DATE DUE

SEP 2 7 2007	
APR 1 4 2008	

DEMCO, INC. 38-2931

Practicing Medicine Without a License!

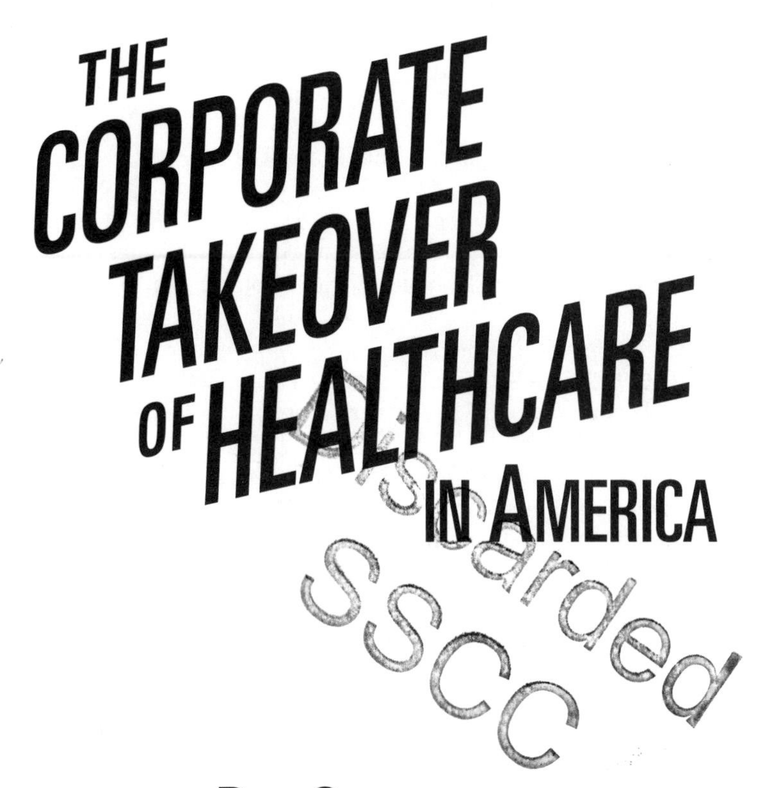

DON SLOAN, MD
with Robin Feman

CAVEAT PRESS
ASHLAND, OR

Caveat Press
PO Box 3400
Ashland, OR 97520
www.caveatpress.com

Cover by David Ruppe, Impact Publications
Interior by Christy Collins

Printed in the United States

Library of Congress Cataloging-in-Publication Data

Sloan, Don M., 1928-
Practicing medicine without a license : the corporate takeover of healthcare in America / by Don Sloan, with Robin Feman.
p. ; cm.
ISBN-13: 978-0-9745245-4-2 (pbk.)
ISBN-10: 0-9745245-4-9 (pbk.)
1. Medical economics. 2. Medical care, Cost of. I. Feman, Robin. II. Title.
[DNLM: 1. Health Care Reform--United States. 2. Delivery of Health Care--economics--United States. 3. Drug Industry--economics--United States. 4. Insurance Coverage--organization & administration--United States. 5. Managed Care Programs--economics --United States. 6. Physician-Patient Relations--United States. 7. Quality of Health Care--economics--United States. WA 540 AA1 S535p 2006]
RA410.58.S66 2006
338.4'33621--dc22

2006019238

As long as one person in the world goes without healthcare, we all do.
To those in need, I dedicate *Practicing Medicine Without a License.* ♦

CONTENTS

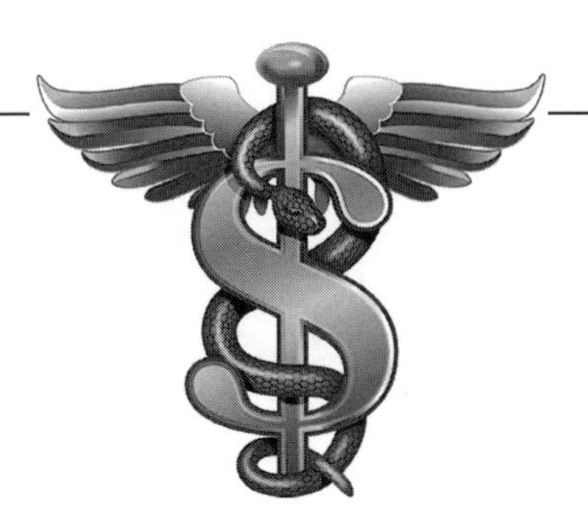

CHAPTER ONE

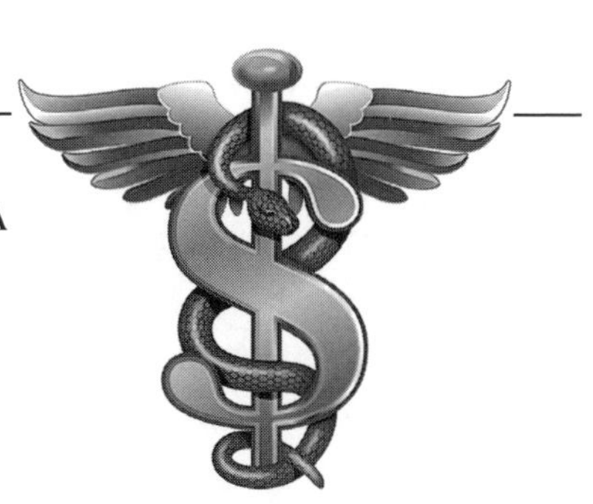

The Wake-Up Call—Jessica and the Doctor Take on the System

I turned the corner, automatically following the city streets to the hospital. There had been many nights like this for me, freezing, dark Sundays, walks on the empty avenues, odd moments of unexpected solitude in the tumult of New York City. Rarely could I appreciate the quiet and peacefulness of my neighborhood while moving toward whatever challenges faced me in the emergency room. Tonight was no exception. My patient, Jessica Riggins, was in distress, perhaps anticipating the emergency surgery we had been trying to avoid.

Earlier in the evening, she had called my answering service with "a real problem that won't let up." Not prone to exaggeration, Jessica was measured in her responses to my findings and analytical in her approach to treatment. She was a woman very much in touch with her health, and although she always went for the "wait and see" attitude, she was not going to ignore me and my concerns foolishly. For her to call me on a weekend meant she was in real trouble.

A return call confirmed my suspicions. She sounded scared. She was scared. "It's really coming down. I'm bleeding through the napkins and may have to use a towel. We don't know what to do." She recounted the sudden pressure and cramps she felt and the outpouring of vaginal blood that had sent her into bed. Although she remained calm on the surface, it was obvious that she was surprised by the sudden hemorrhage. She and her husband, Richard, lived just out of town, and their journey from the 'burbs could take an hour, depending on bridge traffic. I assured her I would be standing by.

As the familiar bright lights of the emergency room rose up in front of me, I was turning another corner still, one I couldn't yet see. It was the beginning of a new and unwelcome chapter in my thirty-five-year career as an obstetrician and gynecologist. Over those decades, I had relied on my own and my colleagues' experience, education, and judgment in caring for my patients. I was therefore wholly unprepared for the new priorities set forth by the managed care industry that had recently taken charge of medicine in the USA and had been creeping up on me slowly but surely. The transition hadn't hit me yet. There are completely different expectations put upon physicians in these times, and they have little to do with the Hippocratic Oath. I was about to learn this the hard way.

As a patient, Jessica Riggins was no different from many others. But she became a catalyst and an ally, and in that, she was far more important to me than I could have expected. Through her, I was forced to understand and accept what I had apparently tried to ignore. My medical practice was being quietly taken away from me, slowly and legally. I was losing control over my patients' treatment plans, becoming simply the middleman between the sick and vulnerable and the insurance companies seeking to elicit whatever financial gains were possible from this suffering.

Without being given a choice, I was an accomplice to this deceit, to my detriment and that of the people who trust me. Less and less each day was I entitled to make those subtle decisions that define quality medical care, decisions made on a case-by-case basis for each individual who believes that this is how I and my colleagues practice medicine. I had been rolling with the tide. The turnover was smooth and steady. It was about to hit me. I was about to become enlightened.

Trust now no longer plays such a large part in our healthcare system. Patients' desires and doctors' judgments are irrelevant as doctors become accountable to groups of off-site strangers whose only interest is in the cost of treatment and the time it takes to move the assembly line along. And, although the physician's freedom to administer care has been greatly diminished by taking on this stealthy "associate," it is he alone who is responsible when a situation takes a negative turn. Whether or not it is his fault, the doctor pays the ultimate price, legally, personally, and financially, through litigation and frustration. This deeply flawed HMO system has crept into our lives without our realizing the power it seeks to control or the damage it inflicts upon healthcare as a whole and the lives of individuals.

I had inherited Jessica's case from my office mate and colleague, Ben Harley, who moved on into semi-retirement in his hometown of Miami. Although Jessica regretted that she had to change doctors, she knew Ben would pass her on to someone trustworthy and personable. Indeed, we hit it off from the start. Her awareness and participation in her own healthcare made for the kind of patient every good doctor seeks and appreciates. Over time, as I proved myself to this bright and discerning woman, she responded with a loyalty and faith that we both found rewarding.

A Good Patient

When we first met, JR, as she liked to be called, was nearly forty-eight years old and the mother of three boys, fourteen to eighteen. She exhibited an understated elegance and sense of fun with fashion, and her fabulous dark brown hair, swinging stylishly above her shoulders, made her appear years younger. Knowing and happy her child bearing years were over, she had recently become quite involved in athletics, joining her husband on the tennis court and golf links. They continued to enjoy spending more time together and looked forward to their quickly approaching twenty-fifth wedding anniversary.

Their marriage was stable and happy, and Jessica commented to me that she was expecting something quite wonderful to celebrate this occasion, and was planning a great surprise for her adored husband. They found themselves doing more and more together. Like daily grocery shopping. Occasionally, when his workday schedule allowed, Dick joined Jessica for her office visits with me. We spent a pleasant amount of time discussing sports, business, and politics—in addition, of course, to his wife's health.

JR started skipping periods a few years after I took over for Ben, but soon, her endocrine system changed its routine. Her periods were sometimes quite heavy and then less regular. A clot or two appeared on occasion, and a sonogram at that time showed the accelerated enlargement of several muscular fibrous tumors, budding on almost all surfaces of her womb.

Years before, in the early stages of their growth, Jessica had been reassured that these "fibroids" were under control, and they could potentially become dormant if menopause came around at an opportune time. In her case, the sooner the better. But her youthful appearance was also indicative of her reproductive status. Menopause was not going to figure into this equation. It was years away yet.

I offered my opinion and words of caution. Since I had already dismissed a malignancy conversion as a very small statistical possibility, Jessica and I spoke of the possibility of hysterectomy down the road. We agreed that if it came to that, it would be better to schedule it at our mutual convenience, rather than risk an emergency procedure. Rushing often causes unnecessary and avoidable complications, I explained. With a planned surgery, I could choose the right timing for her body, the right hour, the right assistants, the right nurses, and the right anesthesiologist. The right everything.

Knowing all that, she still said sweetly, "Let's see what happens next year." It was the same gentle command she had offered following all of her checkups with me over the past three years. She felt healthy otherwise and was not about to rush into major surgery. She glided out the door to her next activity. I instructed her to note the severity of her symptoms and to continue her regular appointments. An annual mammogram was included. JR had an aunt who had succumbed to breast cancer. But, thus far, she had coped quite well with any changes in her body, and she had agreed to remain alert to any warning signs. The next two office visits repeated this pattern of her updates and calm decisiveness, and we waited. It added up to two more "Let's see what happens next year."

Next Year Happened

Finally, there was an abrupt and unpleasant change. The fibroids were making their presence known quite loudly, and Jessica was not happy about suffering the greater inconvenience of the gnawing pain and unpredictable blood flow. I became concerned. Jessica was starting to produce more estrogen than expected, and I didn't know where it was coming from. Her cell smears and blood levels indicated something volatile and erratic was occurring.

The tumor growth was flaring up, and I had to let her know that, at the very least, the size could interfere with her vanity if left untreated. In fact, a little bulge might show through her proudly worn tennis gear, and there was no question what it would be. I detailed my examination thoroughly, but Jessica again insisted that her life not be interrupted. "Let's see what happens next year," was still her final word on the subject. I had expected her reticence. Knowing what I was up against, as long as she didn't bleed outrageously and her blood counts stayed in the normal range, I was comfortable enough to let her ride the wave a little while longer.

Tonight, four months later, the wave knocked her down.

Hospital Time

I was expecting the slippery winter weather and approaching holidays to create an increase of traffic in the ER. Fender benders, falls, scrapes, and bruises were the order for December, when city folks as well as tourists were rushing about in the excitement of the season. Yet, the emergency services were surprisingly quiet, and I didn't have to pull too many strings to move Jessica to the front of the ER line. We quickly fought our way past the triage area to the gynecologic examining section. One look at her face told me that she had lost considerable blood, one feel of her abdomen and palpation of her pelvis told me the rest. The uterus was no longer whispering of trouble—it was screaming out loud.

Fortunately, for the moment, the flow quieted down enough to allow a nurse to draw some blood specimens and set the intravenous line. The staff knew me well, and we worked as a team. Jessica's fear was placated by the cooperative and competent feeling in the room, and things moved quite smoothly. She, Richard, and I made comforting small talk as we waited for the lab to spit out some test results. They told me bad things were happening. Jessica's blood count was half of her last low normal count. The rest of the studies confirmed changes in her metabolism as a result of this blood loss; every system in the human body is interconnected, and when one fails, the others pay a price.

I laid the lab printout on Jessica's lap, and she lifted it from the hospital gown and passed it to her husband without a glance. Of course, they didn't fully understand what they were reading. They left the lab gibberish up to me. They both knew what was going to happen. It was surgery time. Jessica looked at Richard and then me, and said, "Looks like next year is here."

By this time, it was late in the evening. I quickly considered how best to proceed. As qualified as my hospital was to handle the worst-case scenario, I still preferred preparation. I wanted to buy another several hours of time so that I could put the surgery at the top of the morning schedule. Serendipitously, there had been a cancellation that allowed me just that privilege. A call to the operating room alerted the staff to the pending major procedure and the likelihood of a blood transfusion, plus the necessity of all the other precautions for anesthesia when the patient's blood levels could fluctuate suddenly to critical. What we needed now was Jess' cooperation and patience. That I could count on. But we also had to have a hand from Mother Nature. That often wasn't the case. Murphy's Law was hospital gospel. What could go wrong, would. There has never been a single case in any doctor's career that he or she didn't hope to "break the law."

I called for a second blood count, and it showed enough stability to allow for the delay. Her vital signs were also in a safe range, and the hemorrhage was seemingly under control. I told the Rigginses that we'd get Jessica a room, maybe even a sip of apple juice to refresh her, and that she should rest until early the next morning. It was now about eleven in the evening. As the orderlies started transporting Jessica to her room, I instructed Dick to head for the admitting office on the floor above and get through the bureaucratic morass of the admissions process.

I cracked a smile when I warned him that he should be prepared to sign his name dozens of times. He knew what I meant. I took a deep breath, hit the water cooler, and then made the perfunctory required admission call to the 800 toll-free line on Jess' insurance ID card before heading out the door back home, only minutes away. I had several patients on the verge of labor, and I was hoping my phone wouldn't ring tonight in the wee hours for an impending labor and delivery. I wanted to get some shut-eye before my early morning operating room date with Jessica Riggins.

Operating Room Time

I had no sooner taken my second sip from a cup of very inviting hot tea when the phone blared. It had that urgent sound. My resident assistant was about to leave Jessica's bedside when she told him of feeling "wet all over again," and a fast peek revealed the sheets turning red. A stat serum hemoglobin count showed another sharp drop to just over five, meaning Jess had less than half of her normal blood volume. Not acceptable. I told him to cancel the sip of juice and alert the OR we were going to work right now. It was emergency hysterectomy time.

By the time we had one unit of red blood cells piped into JR's veins and optimal anesthetic stability, it was closing in on midnight. I made my incision, opened up Jessica's abdomen, found the expected large and irregular fibroids, and carried out the hysterectomy. My on-duty-by-chance anesthesiologist was fortunately someone I might have even chosen in the morning, and the procedure went strictly according to plan. As much as they ever do.

Jessica rolled into the recovery room just before 2:30AM and was back in her room a bit before noon on Monday. I completed my morning activities and reached Jessica's room on rounds later that afternoon. She was groggy but awake and trying to do more than she should, exactly as I imagined she would, knowing her as I did. Dick was at her bedside. They were obviously relieved they had finally put all of this behind them.

I began my surgical rounds Tuesday morning at 8AM. Jessica was propped up in bed when I arrived and had even urinated without the catheter after being assisted in the walk to the bathroom. She had almost a phobic resistance to bedpans, so I knew she would try this move if at all possible. Fear and a determination to heal were not, however, the only reasons for this show of strength. There are no empty spaces inside the human body. Everything is filled up with organs that fit in just right, just as our maker put us together. So the sizable uterine tumor had therefore impinged on her intestines, causing her abdominal uneasiness over the years that she had ignored. Or just denied. My intraoperative procedure had therefore involved some GI manipulations. That problem, as well, was relieved by the operation.

We were waiting for a return to normal bowel functioning as an indication of a successful recovery. Jess was going to taste food better, digest it better, eliminate it better. The toe bone and head bone are connected. Dragging around an unwanted tumor, however benign, takes its toll on human well-being in many subtle ways. You never know how bad off you were until it all gets relieved, and the comparison is startling. Jessica's prognosis for the second half of her life was excellent.

Daily blood counts would monitor her post-surgery return to normal levels, and I anticipated a steady course from here. But JR had made one trip too many to the bathroom already and suddenly felt too tired to move. With her blood count such as it was, it didn't surprise me at all that her energy was sporadic at best. I convinced her to stay put for a while, and she even agreed to a bedside commode or even that dreaded bedpan until the following morning. Obviously, Jessica's energetic personality was betraying her. The healing process is demanding. She wasn't quite ready for all of this. Major surgery just "ain't for sissies," she said, stealing a line from movie legend Bette Davis about growing old.

On Wednesday morning, Jessica indulged in the hospital's liquid breakfast. "Hospitals must have stock in apple juice companies," JR mumbled with a forced smile. She was excited to report to me that she had checked off yet another step in the recovery process. I congratulated her on the progress, adding a reminder to "take it easy" as I headed for the door. My schedule had me in a rush that day, and after those early rounds at the hospital, I arrived in my office just before eleven to find a full waiting room there, as well.

The HMO Shows Up

As I read through the day's agenda and some patient reports, my intercom signaled a call from a Ms. Maria Lester from Consolidated Insurance Company. It was Jessica's carrier. We exchanged the usual morning greetings and identification data and got down to business. She had been assigned the Jessica Riggins case.

"How is Mrs. Riggins this morning?" I reached for Jessica's office chart in my post-op patient file, prepared for detailed queries about her condition. I knew to sound informed and compliant. I really had no idea what was coming.

"Was she discharged this morning?" asked Nurse Lester.

"No," I replied in a guarded tone. "She might be ready tomorrow, although I think Friday is more realistic. Mrs. Riggins hasn't quite got all her wits about her yet. But she is getting there." I was trying my best to make it sound as though we were in this together and both wanted the best care for "our" patient. I sensed that to Consolidated and Ms. Lester, JR was just another policy holder. A client. A customer.

"Well, it is her third day post-op, and that is her allowance for a hospital stay. Any problem that would delay it after today, doctor?"

I did some quick arithmetic in silence and came up with a different number. "No, Ms. Lester, Mrs. Riggins has only been in her room for two days. Tuesday and today, correct?"

"No, doctor, there is also Monday. That makes three."

Now I knew where she was coming from and where she was going. "Oh, yes," I said with an agreeable air. "But Monday was really the day of surgery. We didn't get started until darn near midnight, so Sunday doesn't count, right?" I used "darn" instead of the harsher-sounding "damn," though I really felt my point cried out for more emphasis. Still, I thought my explanation would suffice and that the debate would end here. No way.

"Doctor, we have her listed as being admitted and into surgery on Sunday. Then there is Monday and Tuesday, and Wednesday is her third day, the day for discharge. Is there any complication that we should talk about?"

I figured I still had a few tricks up my sleeve that were credible. "Well, her vitals are a bit shaky and her hemoglobin count is coming back later this morning. I saw her a couple of hours ago and she still needs some recovery time. Really."

"Well, her temperature is near normal this morning with a normal pulse at 82 and a blood pressure of 118 over 68. Her hemoglobin, let's see here, is at 8.9, up from 7.6 yesterday. That is going in the right direction. Sounds like she is doing nicely."

I had to sit down to finish my conversation. "Run that by me again, please." Ms. Lester did exactly that. The numbers were repeated. "I hadn't gotten the blood counts before I left the hospital this morning, Ms. Lester. How do you know all this?"

"We just pass the patient through our electronic screening units here in the office and get all the info we need, doctor," said Ms. Lester. "And our in-house people tell me she is doing just fine. Your patient should be very grateful, Doctor Sloan." Now Ms. Lester was playing the soft soap game with me. She was being patronizing. I, of course, didn't like how it sounded.

"Where exactly is your office?" I asked. "Where are you calling from?"

"We're in Missouri, not far from downtown St. Louis."

"And you know my patient's vital signs taken in New York maybe a couple of hours ago and her hemoglobin that I haven't even gotten yet this morning? I compliment you on your efficiency. The wonders of technology... Ms. Lester, I saw the patient this morning, and she is just not ready to take on the outside world. She was really doing some heavy bleeding late Sunday and her hemoglobin was near five. That was quite a shock to her system. She will need a day more, at least. I will reevaluate her later on today. Seem right to you?"

"Mrs. Riggins can get some help at home, Doctor Sloan. Housekeeper or family. A visiting nurse service can even come and check up on her. If need be. Whatever. That should do nicely, all part of Consolidated's service and coverage."

There was now silence and I was waiting for the next shoe to drop. I visualized myself going back to the hospital and explaining to Jessica that she had to pack up her toothbrush and head for home. Then I realized I was still in charge of Jessica's care, and that I knew better. Lester was using her technology. I was adding my eyes and ears. "Well, I will talk to the patient and see how she feels about this. May I speak with your supervisor and your medical consultant to explain further?" My resolve was strong. Nurse Lester replied that she would gladly transfer me. "Let me see who is on service today."

A kind sounding older male voice greeted me with a hearty "Good morning. This is Dr. Philip Connor here," but he wasted no time on small talk. He got right down to the business at hand. "Yes, Dr. Sloan," he said, "I looked this thing over, and we are sure that those three days post-op for this healthy woman will be just about right. She sounds like she's in good shape."

I put on my man-to-man, colleague-to-colleague tone, and offered him my now canned lecture about that first day really being near midnight and told him Jessica wasn't ready for discharge. As a fellow clinician, I was sure I could remind him of his own Hippocratic commitment. He wasn't convinced. Turns out he was an old school generalist with some vague obstetric-gynecologic experience over the years who figured that "the lady will be just fine." Now sensing that he had never intended to consider my opinion, I once again agreed to run this by my patient, and hung up the phone. They surely assumed it was a closed matter.

But it was not so for me and Jessica. I sat back in my swivel chair and pondered the creeping realization that I actually was no longer in charge of my patient's care. It was troubling and frustrating, and I was getting angrier by the minute. I didn't quite know yet who was my target. Lester, Connor, Consolidated, my hospital, or just the system. I had to find the right culprit.

I buzzed my waiting room receptionist, Barbara, and told her it would be a few more minutes before I could see the first patient of the day. Then I dialed through directly to Jessica's bedside phone and caught her before her morning exercise, a trip to the window easy chair. There was no need to beat around the bush. I explained the call from Missouri and that her carrier was rather insistent that she leave the hospital today. Perhaps even now. It was perilously close to noon, the witching hour of discharge after which a patient is suddenly fiscally on to the next day. And according to Consolidated, it was a superfluous day. There was silence as she collected her thoughts. I wondered if she understood the nuances of HMO medicine.

"Hold on a minute, Don Sloan," Jessica stammered. "You are the boss. Do you think I should leave right now?"

"No, I don't, Jess," I admitted. "I would like you to hang in here at least one more day, maybe even until Friday. But we have a problem. The long and short of it is, if Consolidated gives us the thumbs down, they won't pay for the time after today, and with your private room rate, you're looking at likely over a thousand bucks a day. It would be your responsibility." I briefly explained to Jessica the way the system handled such situations. I began with the meaning of "carve out," the term coined by insurance companies for denying stays in hospitals they deem unwarranted or excessive.

They simply take note that the patient stayed over her allowed time, that the doctor may have offered a justification and that it was denied. Then they will simply "carve out" those extra days from their reimbursement to the hospital, and the hospital accounts receivable department will send the patient the bill for the difference. This could happen anytime in the future, right on schedule at check out or whenever the auditors get around to it.

She was surprised. I reminded Jessica that hospitals are not exceedingly altruistic, that they are businesses that can be as relentless and ruthless as any when it comes to collections. While it is occasionally true that some people who can afford their bill intentionally deceive hospitals as easily as they do other creditors, that is by far the exception. Yet, those who deserve more sensitive treatment lose out to the cynicism of such potential fraud. Computers and voice mail show no mercy.

Jessica hesitated, a little taken aback. She couldn't believe that we were even debating bureaucratic policy when she had recently endured a major operation that left her feeling as though she had been broadsided by an eighteen-wheeler. She assumed her only concern should be a full recovery in an optimal fashion. I agreed and I again told her so. Adding that she would let Richard know what was happening, JR reminded me that we both already knew that the finances would play no role. Richard would insist that I make the decision that was best for Jessica's health, and he would be willing to either deal with his insurance company later or simply pay the tab. I was happy to have my usual carte blanche with her treatment and figured their priorities into the blueprint. My decision was made. There was no way I was going to discharge my patient that day in her weakened and unstable condition.

JR and I Shake Hands

Jessica was in bed, trying to follow the six o'clock newscast, when I arrived in her room later on in the day. She recounted her activities, and of course, she had been following the doctor's orders to the letter. Her fright with her hemorrhage on the weekend took some of the fight out of her, and I didn't have to say things twice. We went over my conversations with the insurance people, and she again assured me that I was to do what I thought best. Once again, we were in full agreement.

After a restful night's sleep, JR was much more alert during my very early rounds on Thursday. Her last blood count was stable, moving upward, and the nurse on duty reported that Jessica's progress was headed in the right direction. However, she was appearing quite pale and drawn. Walking up and down the hallway on Dick's arm had taken its toll. Sturdy Jessica Riggins had become fragile, and my scalpel didn't help matters.

"I'm staying put today," she immediately remarked. "I couldn't even tie my sneakers the way I feel now. The back nine will just have to wait a while." Another forced smile.

"Sounds right, Jess. Let's shoot for tomorrow. Plan on it."

Later on that morning, after my usual chores at the hospital staff meeting and in the record room, I headed for the office and another call to the HMO offices. After the usual machinations of punching an endless amount of buttons, including my and Jessica's social security numbers and the case record, I waited through the assurances that this was all being done for our security and confidentiality, and was finally promised that someone, a real human being, would be with me shortly. I held on for dear life, hoping that there would be no disconnect that would force me to go through this whole punch-in process again. That had happened to me before. I also hoped that I would reach a department close to the one I sought, if not the exact person supposedly in charge of the case. I counted on hearing Nurse Lester. No such luck.

Finally the live human voice, a very different sounding younger woman, asked for a repeat of the patient's case number and a few minutes to pull up the Riggins file. I assured her that I was happy to continue waiting, as though I had a choice.

She politely gave me her name, but it didn't register. I think I was preparing to get ornery. "How is Mrs. Riggins today, doctor?" came the first question. Now that I knew she already had JR's morning hemoglobin and temperature, I felt somewhat silly giving my report. But I kept my cool and played the game. I needed to buy time for my patient, and I had to be tactful and friendly. I figured that at the first hint of my seeming argumentative, I would be told that a supervisor would take this call and then I would forever be labeled a "troublemaker" in their records. Not to mention, I would have to repeat every detail over again.

"When do you think she will be leaving the hospital, Doctor Sloan?"

I gave the HMO "Provider Services Associate" my instant replay of the case, indicating I would feel secure sending her out in the morning, assuming there were no setbacks.

"Fine, Doctor. I'll mark the file and our committee will review it here next week. Thank you."

By Friday morning, Jessica was obviously more alert and chipper, ready to face the outdoor chill. I remembered being taught that rehabilitation is always better in the spring and summer, so that the patient does not have to tackle the elements as well as her own frailty. For this reason, I was grateful that this post-op patient was now truly physically and mentally ready for the trip home. Relieved, Dick was standing by with an extra blanket and an efficient car heater. Our game plan was to wait out the HMO decision on the two "extra" days Jessica stayed over the allowance, but we all quietly assumed that my resistance had solved the problem. They again both reminded me that I was not to worry about it. I didn't.

At her two- and six-week post-op check-ups in the office, there was only a casual mention of the HMO incident. She had not heard from her insurance company, and the hospital billing rituals had not yet kicked in. The tranquility was broken in late February, about a month later. Richard received a statement from the hospital for those two days in question, for room and board and the minimal medications I had ordered for Jessica's discomfort and sleep. It came to about $2,500. As per our arrangement, he called their accounts receivable department and was told exactly what he had been expecting to hear. The HMO had "carved out" that Thursday and Friday, and the difference was the Riggins' responsibility. I took it from there.

I called the hospital's billing department to let them know the patient was disputing the HMO carve out and that I was in full agreement. I briefly summarized my conversations with the HMO, conscious of keeping my administrators closely informed. My next call was to the Consolidated offices, and again I ploughed through the various computer-generated messages and instructions. I had not yet learned the trick of how to bypass the mechanics of their voice mail system. Taking a deep breath, I promised myself I would keep a level head. But I was prepared for battle.

Getting the Government Involved

It didn't take long to reach that level of discord. After running through the history with yet another Provider Services Associate, I asked for reconsideration of the carve out due to the circumstances. It took until the next day for the HMO supervisor to get back to me and to Richard, informing us that their original decision stood. Again, by our preset arrangement and game plan, we both told Consolidated we were prepared to take whatever steps were needed to make our appeal. I was ready to move forward.

The Blue Pages gave me the number of the local state governmental authorities, and that office provided me with the number of the state insurance control board. I held patiently, finally reaching a contact person who seemed to be knowledgeable. She heard me out and asked that I again detail the events to a colleague of hers who would then be responsible for my case. I was given a number for future reference, and Jessica Riggins vs. Consolidated Insurance Company became No. 66914/MS. I again called my hospital billing department, asking they stand by until the HMO resolved the appeal. They well understood the chronology and workings of the insurance industry.

Later that week, Richard called to assure me that he understood now what I was so worked up over, and although he normally would have paid the bill to avoid a confrontation, this time he would sit back and wait, adding his influence to our struggle. Indeed, the HMO eventually contacted Jessica and Richard, and together they defended our position.

The matter went quietly unresolved. I had received, completed, and filed the necessary papers that documented my complaint. When a call finally came from the state agency regarding case No. 66914/MS, it was late spring. I welcomed a decision, but it was not to be. Things were still up in the air. The HMO had filed a rebuttal in its defense, and I was asked to corroborate my clinical impression that, in view of her condition, Mrs. Jessica Riggins was not ready to leave the hospital that winter Wednesday morning. I reiterated that the first "day" was not more than two hours, despite the quirk of the calendar. I had found a sympathetic ear at the state offices, and they were willing to take it further with Consolidated. I was comforted to have yet another partner in my fight for what was right.

A fly in the ointment rose up when I discovered my hospital, however, was no ally. A staff nursing note described Jessica as "functioning well" on that fateful Wednesday morning, and this simple comment was used to refute my clinical judgment. The sides had been drawn. It was the HMO and the hospital versus patient Riggins and the doctor. We held fast. Weeks passed.

Victory was finally ours. The state insurance board's final telephone call and note indicated that the timing, the pathology, and the clinical events validated my judgment, and the recommendation would be to allow for the extra forty-eight hours. Consolidated, without further ado, acquiesced and paid the piper. The carve out was rescinded. Case closed.

At her semi-annual check-ups, Jessica and I always found time for a little reminiscence and a little gloating. All along, it had seemed like we were David taking on Goliath, and somehow we had won. We had beaten the system. But this taste of victory with the Rigginses was short lived. There came other times when a similar chain of events prompted me to stand up to an HMO, not always with so confident and well-healed a patient and not always with a cooperative state insurance agency.

The Jessica Riggins saga had forearmed and forewarned me that "fighting city hall" is no easy task. But each time I did so in the future, I felt similarly convicted and tried my best to wade calmly through the bureaucratic quicksand to achieve a positive result for my patient. And each time, no matter how justified we were, it was extremely difficult to remain reasonable and maintain my faith in fairness and honor throughout the process of defying our now entrenched healthcare system.

I also subtly felt the sting of my own hospital administration's condemnation. On my semi-annual tally sheet that recorded my bed consumption, I had been red-flagged for using over the mean number of post-op days as stacked up against my colleagues. I was never sure how long it would be before I would get called in to the "principal's" office, forced to stand in the corner, hanging my head in shame.

Over the years, I found myself trading HMO anecdotes with other clinicians, as we topped each other's horror stories of powerlessness and frustration. Every so often, someone at a staff meeting offered the group a variety of tricks and inside tips intended to circumvent the insurance companies' tightfisted approach to medical care. We may have enjoyed these few moments of shared encouragement and hope, but the gloom returned as we heard stories with much less happy endings than Jessica Riggins'. I soberly understood that our small victories were somewhat Pyrrhic. We were winning occasional battles, but quickly losing the war. David would not beat a Goliath who came to the arena wary and prepared.

Winning the Battle, Losing the War

As time goes on, HMO carriers update their rules and regulations, forestalling confrontations with physicians, patients, and local government offices. More and more disclaimers are added annually to the forms that are signed by customers, and these policies take such contingencies as Jessica's into consideration. The fine print gets finer, and the "between the lines" exclusions become more extensive. The insurance companies are protected from every eventuality. Patients and doctors are not.

Understanding that this is the present, I worry about the future. There are millions of Americans who have experienced or will soon experience the aggravation of this process, and some will even suffer physical harm because of it. Until recently, I was unwilling to entertain the possibility of the worse case scenario becoming our only reality, never believing that our healthcare system could fall so short of what it needs to be.

But in truth, it has. As I learn more about how we arrived in this desperate place, I reflect on my earlier oblivion. Could I have foreseen this? Could I have protected other patients? Saved them some heartache when they most needed comfort? Provided stability and guidance when they were being misled and confused?

I don't know exactly when or how I relinquished my judgment and control. The day I finally recognized the vast and irresponsible changes that had altered my medical practice, the shock made it seem like it had occurred overnight. But I know now that it was a gradual process. That I had added a partner to my practice without an invitation became more and more apparent as the years went by. The trouble was that only one of us had a license to practice medicine.

CHAPTER 2

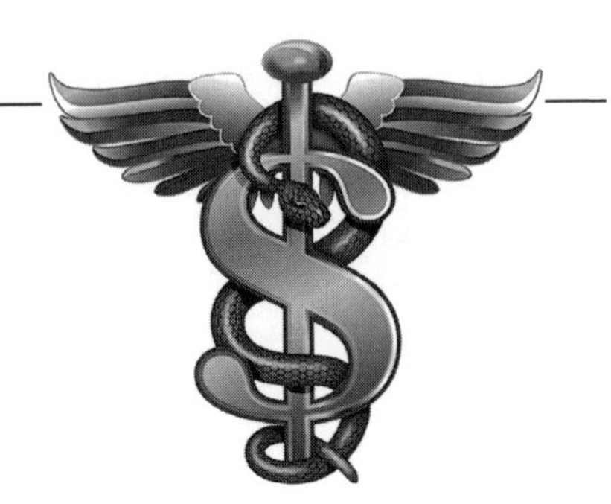

U.S. IS NUMBER ONE! BUT ON WHAT LIST?

Nothing happens in a political vacuum. Nothing. The toe bone is connected to the head bone. Healthcare's place in a country agenda is but a microcosm of where a nation ranks its social consciousness. It reveals the quality of our purpose, our economy, our priorities and where they are placed on the chain of command. Along with education, healthcare tells all about a government and its people.

For without a healthy and literate people, a society cannot succeed. World history has proven that over and over again. Where then does America stand on the ladder of accomplishments when stacked up against the rest of the nations of the world? Sadly, with all of its opulence, power, wealth, and resources, nowhere near high enough.

U.S. FOREIGN AID

For openers, we have often bragged about how generous we are toward the rest of the world as measured by our foreign aid. Politically, it is no secret that we base our aid not on need, but on its service as a tool of our foreign policy. Countries that are friendly to the U.S. power structure are the beneficiaries of our benevolence. Thus, the nations that receive by far the lion's share of our foreign aid are Israel and Egypt, the two nations in the Middle East boiling pot that are most politically aligned with our ideals and ambitions.

If generosity has been properly defined as the giving of what you have little of, then in that context, no matter how benevolent we might seem, we are not a generous nation. Even now, there is that brouhaha over our rehab funding of Iraq. Revelations come daily of contracting through the Halliburton empire and other corporate friends of the

Administration, based not on value or need, but on the size of contributions to the various political campaigns or their political connections.

Despite our reputation, the numbers betray it as false. For although we have been ballyhooed as the world's foremost social worker, the truth is sadly the opposite. The United States of America continues to give less overseas aid as a percentage of its Gross National Product (GNP) and income than any other developed nation. With the exceptions of aid to Israel and Egypt, we allocate and spend more in one day on the military operation in the Gulf War than we spend all year on social foreign aid. Likewise, here at home, the Pentagon spends more in fifteen minutes than is federally funded for women's healthcare in a year! Other similar examples abound.

We fall behind most other industrialized nations in just about every area of social need. In percentage of one-year-old children fully immunized against polio, we are number seventeen. China and even Brazil are in front of us. There are lower rates of low birth weight babies born in Egypt and Jordan than here at home. Before the debacle of 1989 that took away its socialized healthcare, the then-USSR was also ahead of us on that list. Lebanon, Libya, and Cuba have more teachers for their children than the USA.

Oh, yes. We are first among western industrialized nations when it comes to the percentage of children living below the poverty line, murders of males between ages fifteen and twenty-four, in the number of handguns in the street used by people of all ages, the percentage of citizens incarcerated, energy consumption per capita, and in the emissions of air pollutants.

And, we are by far number one in the rate of people gunned down each year in street crimes and similar violent incidents. In America today, there are more African-American adult males in jail than in college.

Shameful Statistics

The World Health Organization (WHO), the arm of the United Nations (UN) that is in charge of the world's state of health, as well as its monitoring and reporting, has often reminded the U.S. that we lag far behind the other G-7 countries, including Australia and Canada, in what the WHO states is "healthy life expectancy." Its latest report suggests that there are many "Third World pockets" within the U.S.

borders. I remind you that over 45 million U.S. Americans have no healthcare coverage at all, and it is easily estimated that over 40 million more have healthcare that can only be described as inadequate. Of course, as expected, much of this follows along racial and ethnic lines, with blacks and Hispanics over-represented among the denied groups.

Life spans alone tell the story. White males are at 75.4 years, white women at 80.5; African-American males hover at 69.2, black women are 76.1. These numbers have improved slightly overall in the past decade, but shockingly are in decline compared to other industrialized nations.

In fact, America sits weakly at number twenty-nine of the thirty-five nations included in the latest UN Human Development Report released in 2005, which lists average life expectancy. It is notable that not only have more countries moved ahead of the USA, but also the gap between us and the healthiest country, Japan, with its average life expectancy of eighty-two years, continues to widen.

The WHO report stated that Native Americans, rural African-American males, and much of the inner city poor have numbers that match many Third World nations. Shamefully, our U.S. is the world's only nation that reports its healthcare statistics in two categories, one for black and the other for white citizens. The differences are that stark.

It has been wisely written that the most heinous and pervasive weapon of mass destruction is poverty. Affluent USA has not escaped that dungeon. Even during our greatest periods of economic boom—strictly subjective depending on who is doing the reporting and whether it is an election year or not—almost one in five (18.5 percent) U.S. children were living in officially defined poverty as we entered the twenty-first century, with black and Hispanic poverty numbers nearly double that of white and Asian. This, despite our gross domestic product's (GDP) nearly doubling in the last quarter of the twentieth century. It is clear that not everyone gets to enjoy the perks of a strong economy. The streets of America that are "paved with gold" are apparently not trod upon or open to all.

UNICEF AND THE U5MR

The United Nations Children's Fund (UNICEF), the UN agency responsible for gauging and recording the medical health of the world's children, has always been seeking the most valid and reflective way to measure. Traditionally, the use of maternal mortality (number of deaths in pregnant women) and infant mortality (either the deaths of neonates within the first twenty-four hours of birth (neonatal mortality) or in the first twenty-eight days of life (perinatal mortality) have been used as the universal barometers. However, as the world has developed in such a drastically broad way, with the richest and poorest nations showing such wide gaps in affluence, these numbers have been shown to be inaccurate and nearly useless in many obvious ways, for various reasons.

First, social structures in the Third World of nations have poor and inadequate means of tabulation. Many parturients give birth outside of hospitals and satellite clinics. Home births or those in the vast wastelands of many undeveloped nations are never counted in the "city hall" of their communities. Moreover, the deaths of these infants at birth, on that first fateful day or during that first month, are also unrecorded, and so are lost to the census takers.

Maternal mortality, once considered a most valid measuring stick, now demonstrates that ever-widening distance between the developed and undeveloped worlds, and only shows a part of the picture. UNICEF-defined, it is "a woman dying during pregnancy or in the process of childbirth," and its inaccuracy stems from the ways the numbers are skewed by circumstances surrounding pregnant women.

For example, as modern highway fatalities are products of various forms of industrialized activity and will rise exponentially according to the numbers of highways, automobiles, as well as the quality of both roadside regulations and highways and themselves, it follows that a more modernized and industrialized society, with its high-speed autobahns and turnpikes, could have a higher rate of maternal mortality.

Racing Maseratis and Porches kill more than plodding burros and galloping llamas. More on-the-job accidents mount up and contribute to mortality overall and thus more maternal mortality. But this would be indicative not of a nation with general poor health or a lack of gestational care and prenatal technology, but of one with more manufacturing plants and advanced consumerism.

This is not to say that both infant and maternal mortality are entirely useless as statistics, only that there is room for improvement. But many other illustrations comparing the lifestyles of the haves and have nots show the folly of those statistics when they are being used to teach and correct. Moving along in the fast lane of life has its drawbacks and risks.

In the early 1990s, UNICEF introduced the under-five-mortality-rate (U5MR), which is currently used by its staff as the latest accepted barometer of a nation's health. Simply defined and applied, its simplicity to its advantage, the U5MR is the number in any given year in any nation of living children at age five per 1,000 births.

With but one number to report, those births unknown or unrecorded to the demographers would be less meaningful statistically. They count on the size of the birth rate and population of living five-year-olds to help to neutralize those that fall through the statistical cracks. Living five-year-olds are more easily traceable and accountable. Lost newborns, for many reasons, are disposed of by grieving families and do not carry the onus of religious, moral, or legal ramifications.

The results immediately bore out the value of the U5MR. It is slowly replacing all other statistics as a reflection of a country's health. Especially when placed alongside other demographics in areas peripheral to healthcare.

The latest *State of the World's Health,* an official UNICEF journal, lists the world's 191 United Nations member countries in order of various achievements and stacks them up using other demographics that are considered meaningful. There are a few surprises.

The best U5MR ratings in 2004, for example, were found in Singapore, Japan, and Scandinavia, followed by countries in Western Europe, Canada, Australia, Cuba, and the United States. They boast numbers in the five to ten range, meaning that for every 1,000 babies born, at least 990 are alive at age five.

An early UNICEF poster shows a smiling Third World little boy with the bottom caption asking, "What do you want to be when you are five?" The second panel shows this same smiling lad, and the caption reads, "Alive!" ♦

To UNICEF, the mark of accomplishment and achievement is a U5MR of fifty. This number has been achieved so far by First and Second World nations with a few exceptions in the Third World. The worst countries are in the range of 250 to 300, meaning that barely 700 children at age five are alive per 1,000 births. Of the worst twenty countries, eighteen are in sub-Saharan Africa. In 2005, the dubious honor of the very worst went to Afghanistan. In the western hemisphere, just about all of South and Latin America are in the 100 to 150 range.

Only three sovereign nations in the Caribbean have broken through and hover at about ten to fifteen: Costa Rica, as evidence to its enigmatic commitment to healthcare despite its impoverished economy; Jamaica, likely from its marked long-standing British influence and occupation; and Cuba, a testimonial to its world-renowned socialized healthcare system that has delivered total healthcare to all its people. It is interesting to note that the USSR, with its almost seventy-five years of socialized medicine, reached a U5MR of thirty in 1990. Since the political changeover in 1991, with a loss of many of its socialized services, it is climbing toward fifty. In the Middle East, Israel stands alone below that magic number.

Other Demographics that Matter

As a way of attesting and confirming the accuracy and value of the U5MR ratings, UNICEF then examined certain other parameters significant in their meanings and merit of a nation's well-being. There were two that matched country for country with the U5MR—percentage of the population with access to potable water and the rate of literacy (defined as a reading ability of at least a ten-year-old). Again, the representative best in both are Singapore, Japan, Western Europe, Canada, Cuba, and the U.S. The worst, as expected, are in sub-Saharan Africa and southern Asia.

As claimed by many world health authorities and confirmed by UNICEF, in order to achieve adequate healthcare for a population, a society must have decent sanitation and education. It has been rightly said that for a people to understand the role of good health, they must have access to drinkable water and the proper sanitation that leads to it, and they must have the ability to follow their doctors' orders and comprehend the need for proper preventive care and treatment prescriptions. The three—healthcare, literacy, and potable water—go hand in hand.

But once again, among all the nations of the UN, only the U.S. must bear the shame of a two-figure report—one for the U.S. black and one for the white population. The circa ten rating achieved by the U.S. for its U5MR has an asterisk attached. For white America the number ranks with the best, less than five. But for its people of color, the U5MR is quadruple that, and thus the reported ten is an average. That is the number that we as a nation must approach, work on, and improve.

Just as a way of comparison, there are those who still report on infant mortality as their gauge of a society's health and have as yet not adopted the UNICEF U5MR scale. The 2004 score as reported in the January 2005 *New York Times* for the Americas has Canada, Cuba, the USA, Jamaica, Costa Rica, and Chile among the best, with the rest of Latin and South America dawdling behind.

On a general world scale, taking all parameters of healthcare into consideration and not only the neonatal and maternal mortality but also cardiac deaths, cancer morbidity, infectious diseases, strokes, and even trauma, the U.S. ranks somewhere about twenty-fifth. That despite our enormous prosperity on so many levels.

There are thus those many other demographics that are all a part of the abysmal state of the U.S. healthcare system. But none is more opprobrious than the present state of poverty in the nation and especially that of child poverty and the condition of the country's children in general. In essence, there is no group in our social order that is more victimized from our lack of healthcare than our children—the group without voting power or a voice of their own. We must speak for them.

It was Senator Kay Bailey Hutchison (R-TX) who said from the floor of Congress that our sad state of healthcare is exhibited in the growing rate of child poverty in the nation. As so stated by the Senator and using U.S. Department of Commerce and Agriculture statistics, the child poverty rate rose to 17.6 percent and in women rose to 12.4 percent in 2004.

U.S. Poverty Rates

With these burgeoning numbers, perhaps it is not a surprise—though it should be a shock—that the U.S. poverty rate for children is *double* that of any country in the developed world. The number of U.S. citizens lacking medical health insurance goes hand in hand and is up by over one million each and every year. That translates to over 15 percent of our population, despite our being "the beacon to the world."

Since we have those over 45 million without any coverage and another 40-plus million with inadequate care, the respected Commonwealth Fund (CF) has stated that, despite some successes along the way, "American children largely don't get the quality of healthcare they should." The Fund added that up to three-quarters of American children do not get the care that would be considered anywhere near optimal.

Certain conditions with readily available treatments are not universally managed. Worse, some of these pathologies are amenable to preventive care. The CF report stated that, for one example, only one-third of children who need asthma control medications ever get them. Over three-quarters of sexually active adolescents with exposure to the easily controlled sexually transmitted disease (STD) chlamydia ever get tested or treated.

Key vaccines might never reach their human targets, even though readily available and affordable, often due only to inadequate Congressional attention. Some years ago, in the early 1990s, as the AIDS epidemic was reaching its peak in the USA, Congress debated a very controversial HIV clinic-funding bill. It failed to get a needed majority for a variety of political, social, and fiscal reasons.

But attached was a rider that allocated some 9 million dollars to complete measles vaccinations for every child in America. That reported year, there were thirty infant AIDS deaths stemming from mothers infected with the HIV syndrome. But, and quickly stonewalled to avoid embarrassment, there were as well thirty very avoidable deaths in children from ordinary variola (measles), endemic in U.S. society. Shocking and shameful, but true. How could this ever happen in affluent America?

The answer lies in priorities. To deny funds for AIDS newborns is to put the onus on the parturients out of their own negligence and irresponsibility in a cruel blame-the-victim game. But to admit to that funding gap for the variola was to have to fess up to their Congressional indifference.

The states in general, including the so-called advanced states in the Northeast, still do not have vaccination programs for all children because of a shortage of federal matching funds—and that lack of priority.

The CF reported that 79 percent of our emotionally disturbed and dysfunctional youth in America were either never seen in consultation at the onset of their mental illness or never had imperative follow-up care.

These disgraces are time bombs waiting to explode.

In *The Progress of Nations*, UNICEF felt obligated to single out the U.S. for its lack of delivering health and support care to its young people. It reminded the world body of nations that as we went through the last decade of the twentieth century, the rest of the industrialized world, through their healthcare packages, became more generous to their children, while the United States became less so.

The UN agency added that some of the young people of color in the inner cities of the U.S. have less sanguine statistics than those in South Africa. Perhaps it is no wonder that administration after administration in Washington have defended their laxity in paying up their UN dues by citing what they consider to be unfair treatment by both UNICEF and other UN reporting agencies. Why feed the mouth that bites you?

Closer to Home

During the Bush *pére* Administration, the federal government issued an embarrassing report that noted forty states failed to spend almost $2 billion, 45 percent of just over $4.2 billion allocated by Congress to the fifty states for children's healthcare programs. California and Texas, President Bush *fils*' home state, accounted for over half of the unspent monies, about $500 million each. Together, these two states have 29 percent of the nation's almost 12 million uninsured children. That number increased as well during the eight years Bill Clinton was in the Oval Office.

Even the poorest states, mostly in the South, did not dispense all of their federal matching funds for children's healthcare. Florida, West Virginia, and even Illinois and New Hampshire, along with several others, had leftover money that was therefore lost, since the regulations call for the return to the federal coffers if not spent within a certain defined time period.

When spokespersons for Governor Jeb Bush of Florida were asked to explain this ignominious action, the reply indicated only that "... there was a lag in getting the programs up and started." I leave it to your imagination to wonder if a "lag" would be tolerated when defense contractors in these same states are to be awarded lucrative and usually unbid-on arms contracts.

Using infant mortality figures as a guide, America's flagship city, New York, reported that 2003 saw a reverse in the positive trend and a rise instead almost across the board for infant deaths in each of the five boroughs. In the Bronx and in Manhattan above the 96th Street parallel, there was the sharpest increase, surely a fallout of the curtailments of Medicaid coverage for many inner city people who were cut from the rolls after two years, based on unemployment and welfare entitlement in the years since the Reagan Administration cuts in the 1980s.

The U.S. Census Bureau's latest report compared American kids against the rest of the developed world nations. It was not our proudest moment, to be sure. Child poverty rates put Russia and the U.S. at the top (worst) and the expected Scandinavia and the rest of Western Europe at the bottom—the best. The U.S. was Number One! in the single-mother household poverty rate.

We are near the worst in public spending on primary and secondary education as a percentage of the GNP, and as expected, the U5MR, although at a respectable combined black and white eightish, is almost double that of Japan, Sweden, and Germany, all with nationalized healthcare coverage for everyone.

Among U.S. working people, ostensibly with a living wage, healthcare stands alone as their severest deprivation. As NAFTA, CAFTA, LAFTA (North American, Central American, and Latin American Free Trade Agreements), and other World Trade Organization (WTO) pacts fall into place, U.S. workers are seeing their jobs shipped abroad, and the domestic U.S. wages that we do get to hang onto do not keep pace with even a seemingly well-controlled inflation. In fact, real wages, those based on inflation and cost of living increases of all sorts, keep falling. In 2004, the rate of decline even increased.

Management at the highest levels and executives in all major U.S. industries are seeing wages and severance benefits and packages rise at twenty to thirty times higher than those on the line. Indeed, if the mass working minimum wage would keep pace with management, the present $5.15 would now be at over $15. Moreover, the U.S. worker has the longest workweek and less vacation time of any counterpart in the industrialized world.

Life Spans

Longevity, also a time-honored benchmark for health status and as well a reflection of a nation's U5MR, has also slipped from the hands of citizens in the U.S. Yes, American life spans of the white population climbed past the seventy-five-year mark as we entered the twenty-first century, but remember that white and black still show their usual gaps.

Thus, with our combined average, we lag behind all of Western Europe, Israel, Canada, Australia, and even some parts of Eastern Europe that were formerly within the Soviet bloc, and certainly Japan, which this past year enjoyed its status as number one on the United Nations U5MR tables. No, we are not at the ugly level of the barely forty years that a child in Sierra Leone and much of Africa faces at birth, but we are a far cry from the eighty-two years expected by all Japanese citizens.

African-American male life spans still have not reached even seventy-five years, due to a relentless AIDS death rate, untreated cardiovascular conditions, lung cancer, and violence. UNICEF has stated that nine out of ten young people slain in industrialized nations are Americans here at home. The U.S. homicide rate for people ages fifteen to twenty-four is five times that of its nearest competitor, Canada.

The Population Reference Bureau (PRB), a Washington private demographic organization, compiles these statistics regularly. Its think tanks have also noticed and publicized that the U.S. numbers suffer in comparison to the rest of the industrialized world because of the abysmally lower figures for the 25 percent of the U.S. population who come from so-called minority groups. The international medical literature is constantly watching over our shoulders and continually chides the U.S. for its failure to deliver proper healthcare to everyone.

The prestigious Institute of Medicine, commenting on the state of U.S. healthcare during the 2004 presidential campaign, pointed out that the weaknesses of the Bush II Administration were in areas of social policy of all sorts, with healthcare failures leading the way. It is no wonder that all candidates for just about any level of office felt compelled to issue some sort of disclaimer, as though to distance themselves from the terrible federal policies that don't give us healthcare.

Our failure to be the very best in this social area has not escaped medical-politico thinkers, even those who are traditionally aligned with the establishment and the status quo in Washington. Doctor Arnold S. Relman, Professor Emeritus at Harvard and former editor of the revered *New England Journal of Medicine (NEJM),* broke ranks and labeled our system far from Number One; he called it "expensive, inefficient, and inequitable." Doctor Relman's remarks were made in front of the right audience—a U.S. Senate committee on Social Affairs, Science and Technology. He added that our dearth of healthcare delivery was all the more blasphemous since we continually boast of our technical and scientific accomplishments. He did not pull any punches, telling the committee that our private medical system with (sic) profits put before people was at the basis for a failure to deliver the care to people that we learned in our laboratories and research centers. That "for profit" HMO system has failed.

The distinguished Commonwealth Fund also found it necessary to reprimand our authorities for their disregard of our healthcare system after its review of over 150 studies and reports on that status. "Substandard and...disparities" in care were at fault.

The National Academy of Sciences also jumped on the bandwagon, forced to admit that we are certainly not where we should be when it comes to healthcare.

"Being uninsured can be bad for your health," it stated.

Interruption of medical insurance, when those covered are dismissed or lose their jobs for whatever reason, is devastating. Most often, the affected cannot fall back on the continuation of the allegedly purposeful benefits act (COBRA) because of the costs involved, which start out at several thousands of dollars a year, well beyond the reach of just about all the unemployed. Doctor Relman reiterated the problem—a for-profit healthcare system that puts profits before people.

The Numbers Tell the Story

Other numbers and statistics belie the sad truth and tell the sad story. Administrative costs of our present systems are double and even triple those of other comparable countries. Whereas Canada, the UK, and the other members of the G-7, with some form of nationalized health coverage, pay in the range of 5 percent for the bureaucratic machinery to run their systems. The U.S. costs are and were never less than a stated 14 percent. In some areas, costs are as high as 20 percent. The noted exceptions are Medicare and Medicaid, the two federal healthcare programs now operating, which have kept their bureaucracy below 5 percent, where it should be.

One of the most glaring gaps in the U.S. system is among the working poor, dispelling the myths that healthcare holes are relegated to the unemployed, the derelicts, the homeless, and the disheveled and disenfranchised.

It is almost a given that only two-job families can barely afford the private coverage available to most Americans. Historically, one partner might have been in a union and received healthcare benefits this way, but now less than 15 percent of U.S. workers are unionized, well down from the heyday of the 1940s and during World War II when about one-third of the work force were members of some form of representative labor organization.

Unions wanting to regain their lost ground still use healthcare as an enticement. In spite of the fact that it has obviously not been enough to maintain their numbers—the trade union as a group has been reluctant to join to clamor for universal healthcare. Enigmatically, they fear that if there is an affordable and adequate healthcare program available to all American citizens, they cannot dangle this as a perk specific to union membership, thus making that membership less attractive. They would have to find another draw. So, in what can only be seen as against their best interests, they refuse to budge from their position to use the strength of the numbers they still hold in the fight for universal healthcare.

Another well-publicized instance of the working people being unfairly treated and financially disadvantaged in the name of healthcare has received a great deal of media attention, because the main player is the nation's largest employer, Wal-Mart. This retailing behemoth, the biggest business in the world, with operations worldwide in Europe, South America, and Asia—and reported sales in 2004 of over $285 billion—essentially offers no healthcare coverage to its mainline employees. There are loopholes galore, mostly based on its intricate part- and full-time work status.

For a Wal-Mart employee on the line making about $16,000 a year in gross pay, a contributory form of healthcare is offered for over $40 weekly, including dental, coming to almost $3,000 annually. It should come as no surprise that less than half of Wal-Mart workers can take on such coverage. There is noise now being made, with Maryland leading the way, to enact legislation to force Wal-Mart into allocating a minimum percent, now set at eight, of their gross net sales toward employee healthcare coverage. Wal-Mart had set the example; other major employers followed suit. The workers are proffered a combination of retirement plans, such as the 401K with health coverage, which sounds appetizing. A bad taste in the mouth is what it is.

Costs of Healthcare Hit Home

In order to study the relative comparisons between those developed nations with a single-payer, government-sponsored program and the U.S., expenses per person have as well been tabulated. The Kaiser Family Foundation in California recently completed an analysis of this issue, starting with Medicare and Medicaid data and then compiling statistics from the U.S. private healthcare carriers.

In 1990, an annual average of $2,738 was spent on healthcare for every U.S. citizen. By 2004, it had reached close to $6,200 for that same coverage per capita, overtaking expected inflationary allowances. This is more startling when compared to the same numbers for Great Britain and Canada, for example, with their national health services (NHS) at about $2,000. Always be mindful that these nations boast similar or better U5MRs and other healthcare demographics than the United States.

Healthcare costs are indeed rising faster than incomes. Health insurance premiums paid into the coffers of the private carriers in the U.S. have risen three times faster than the average earnings over these past five years, eroding the incomes of average Americans. The Kaiser numbers and published federal data are in agreement.

Another way of looking at the costs of healthcare coverage in comparable industrialized nations is to rate them as based relative to the GNP, the total figure representing the worth of any nation as measured by the total costs of all sales and purchases of all goods and services.

Although all nations show rising costs of healthcare as a part of the GNP, it is indicative of our failings here at home when we see that the nations with federally run programs have better figures than ours. The United Kingdom and Japan hover around 6 percent; Canada at 8 percent; Germany just under 10 percent; the United States is now at 14 percent with a projection of over 16 percent by the years 2008–10.

These other countries have managed to stem the tide of costs while achieving near universal coverage. This takes into account the differences among these other industrialized nations: France and Italy are decentralized but with strong provincial control, all dependent and responsible to their national center; Japan, the present U5MR leader, exists under a more privatized system but with very strong national commitments and regulations.

What is facing America was clearly reported in the *Journal of the American Medical Association (JAMA)* at the beginning of this millennium, in a list "documenting the tragedy of the traditional medical paradigm."

It noted that the yearly 250,000 iatrogenic ("induced by a physician") deaths is the third leading cause of death in the U.S., after cardiac diseases and cancers.

The list looked like this:

- Unnecessary surgery 12,000
- Medication errors in hospitals 7,000
- Other errors in hospitals 20,000
- Infections in hospitals 80,000
- Non-error, negative effects of drugs 106,000.

The report said the U.S. had 116 million "extra" patient visits, 77 million unused prescriptions, 17 million emergency room visits, 8 million hospitalizations, and 3 million long-term admissions.

This might all be tolerated if it resulted in better health, but the report asked, does it? In *JAMA's* comparison of thirteen countries, the United States rates an average second from the bottom on the list of available health indicators, as follows:

- 13th for low birth weight percentages
- 13th for low neonatal and infant mortality
- 11th for post-natal mortality
- 10th for age-adjusted mortality
- 10th for life expectancy at fifteen for females
- 12th for life expectancy at fifteen for males
- 10th for life expectancy at forty for females

- 9th for life expectancy at forty for males
- 3rd for life expectancy at eighty for females and males
- 5th in alcohol consumption

In recent years, the U.S. has boasted of a leveling off of the relative costs of healthcare to GDP as a testament to the workings of the HMO privatized system we are now under. The *JAMA* report, of course, omits our relentless lack of coverage for everyone, the tens of millions of Americans who see no relief in sight.

We cannot rest and or put this aside until we are number one on every one of these parameters. We have the vast and remarkable resources to pull this off. Our work is cut out for us.

Effects on Women and the Poor

Another segment of our American society that has suffered in a unique way without healthcare coverage is numerically a majority but treated as a minority: women. This is telltale in many obvious and also subtle ways.

The furor these past thirty-plus years over abortion/choice, ever since the landmark 1973 Roe v Wade decision and even before the time when various states enacted their own choice statutes, has seemingly ignored the fact that this issue is as volatile as it is, in part, because it affects that particular group—women.

There is no counterpart procedure in the male, of course, by nature or physiology, but making women a target for any type of deprivation is an easier task than it would be for men. Choice would not hold the place it does in our thinking and political arena, despite its religious and moral issues, had women as a whole always enjoyed the total and the full healthcare they deserve.

The Centers for Disease Control (CDC) has included this interpretation in measuring perinatal mortality as a result of prematurity and low birth weight newborns. These have long been attributed, in the main part, as a result of inadequate prenatal care, specifically a need of females, and is something that has been confirmed throughout the world. The CDC has made the suggestion again and again that the impoverished regions of the globe and also the U.S. have sparse prenatal facilities, allocating an inordinate portion of their budgets to the more dramatic treatment of cardiac states and cancers—conditions that are more common in the male population.

There are direct demographic associations between low-income women and the uninsured, access to prenatal care, and in the final picture, care in general. A scale devised by the Kaiser Family Foundation compared women who were uninsured to those on Medicaid and those with private full coverage. Three areas were studied in particular to support their conclusion that a denial of prenatal care led to greater perinatal and neonatal morbidities, as expected. Thus, the U.S. numbers were significant. Medical case records for well care, routine breast exams, and PAP smear visitations were examined. It was clear from the study that the uninsured were the least attended to, by more than double the others. Then came the Medicaid group, followed by the best cared for—the privately insured.

In another subtle indictment of the attitude toward healthcare for women, the Kaiser Foundation survey reported the differences in dealing with female patients *vis à vis* the newly approved French RU-486 abortifacient pill. Less than half of the ObGyns and less than one-third of the family practitioners would eventually be able to offer this management to their women patients. Its medical pros and cons are not being debated—only its availability.

The New York City Department of Health and Mental Hygiene's latest report echoed the KFF with its opening headline: many New Yorkers are not getting the medical care they need. More than 500,000 people in a city of just over 8 million reportedly needed unavailable medical aid. In the eighteen to sixty-four age group, 31 percent have no coverage at all, twice the rate of the publicly insured and six times that of those with private insurance. One out of six New Yorkers does not have a doctor they call their own. Having a personal doctor is considered a luxury outside the grasp of those who have to rely on public assistance healthcare coverage.

The differences between the boroughs are stark and mirror the rest of U.S. inner cities. While fewer than 10 percent of the residents of the affluent Upper East Side of Manhattan report their health as poor or fair, over one-third of Bronxites make that claim.

What is the bottom line? The opening line. That nothing happens within a political vacuum. Poor health filters down and erodes a society. When people do not read and write, they seem to lose out on many other necessities and perks of life.

Some years ago, I applied for a grant from the New York State Department of Health to create a medical school-based program to address the various issues that arise during an under-served, welfare-assisted woman's pregnancy that impact her psychological well-being and emotional comforts. In describing these patients' needs, I used the phrase "quality of life" as our goal for improvement.

The ensuing rejection letter stated that while I was being commended for a well-conceived grant proposal with good intent, the department funds could not be designated just to "improve the quality of life." I wonder what would have been the embarrassment if the health authorities realized the sad irony of what they had written. ♦

There is a myriad of data and statistics that tell of the number of people in the U.S. who succumb to preventable diseases and conditions, who are denied the basics of healthcare that are described year after year by every president as he vies for office and promises that the need will finally be addressed and solved. But it never comes to pass.

Those millions of Americans go without coverage at one time or another. Over 10 million of our children never have that security and attention. Each and every year, on each and every campaign whistle stop, the major political parties scream out that they are the ones to finally end that drought. But it never comes to pass.

We see it ignored again and again and then promised again and again by the next inaugural speaker or in the State of the Union address. This time, it will be corrected on his watch. This time, it will be different. "Just wait and see." But it never comes to pass.

How the USA Compares

What is the state of healthcare in the U.S. today? Our USA spends over 50 percent more than say, Switzerland, on healthcare per capita, the country next in line. And on average, we spend 150 percent over other industrialized nations. The number of beds per capita in the U.S. is consistently in the bottom quartile of those countries.

And that filters down to all other healthcare expenses, from hospital overheads to medical malpractice to prescription drugs. The latest data from the Organization for Economic Cooperation and Development

(OECD) has now confirmed what we already knew. The OECD also points out that although the United States spends more, we do not receive the services we pay for.

Healthcare layout accounts for about 15 percent of the U.S. GDP at a time when only two other countries, Switzerland and Germany, put out more than 10 percent. Averaging over the first years of the new millennium, the United States spends circa $5,200 per person on healthcare. Canada $2,900; Germany $2,800; Switzerland $2,600; Britain $2,200. Yet, each of them boasts of a longer life expectancy, lower infant mortality, and better U5MRs than we. All have a national healthcare service that covers all their people. No one is shut out.

The United States has 2.9 hospital beds per 1,000 residents compared with 3.7 beds/1,000 in the average OECD nation; 2.4 physicians per 1,000 people compared to 3.1/1,000; 7.9 nurses/1,000 compared to 8.9/1,000 among the others.

The U.S. has 12.9 CT scanners per one million population compared with 13.3 elsewhere in the developed world. We do have more magnetic resonance imaging (MRI) machines than the other OECD nations listed, but ours are only in use ten hours daily, compared to fourteen in the others.

The Best Healthcare is Available

The OECD conclusion was not a surprise. We just do not get enough for our buck. But that is not true for everyone in the country. There is an employee/insurance deal in the U.S. that includes unlimited doctor office visits of your choosing; covers all accidents, routine exams, physical therapy, labs and X-rays; and the like; unlimited hospital visits and stays; certain chronic care and rehab; full prescription coverage; and unlimited specialty consultations. For the employee and the entire family. There are no deductibles, no co-pays. and only a $35 monthly fee taken from an annual salary of $158 thou. Thirty-five dollars!

The group awarded this insurance looks forward to a full pension and continued coverage until their deaths. Quite a few, most in fact, were millionaires before they took on their jobs that got them such a perk. Who gets this coverage? It would be nice if it were the underprivileged or the chronically ill and debilitated or our veterans.

But no. For starters, the 535 members of the U.S. Congress, and add to that the few hundred in the upper executive and judicial branches of government. They are also members of a demographic group where seven were arrested for shoplifting, nineteen for writing bad checks, and eighty-four for drunk driving. This bunch also has an overrepresentation of felony indictments, and a few ended up serving time.

And, they are also the very same group who keeps such credible healthcare proposals and bills like John Conyers' HR676 and Barbara Lee's HR3000 holed up in committee, year after year, denying them access to a public hearing and floor vote. In 2005, the president and his cronies up on the Hill voted to slash $10 billion over the next decade from Medicaid. Their own medical benefits stayed intact.

Could it be they don't believe that the rest of America should share in what they are so fortunate to have? We know better. That is the kind of care that we should all have and can afford.

A play with the numbers is even more revealing. Using those same governmental accounting sources, the billions spent on the Iraqi campaign yearly would have given similar healthcare benefits to four out of every five Americans for a year. Think about that.

As the denied are reported to number in the many millions, the profits amassed by the pharmaceutical industry and the robber barons that are the insurance and banking healthcare conglomerates are measured in billions. The arguments used in lobbying against the allowance of pharmacy generics that would slash the costs of drugs to a needy people would match the New York State Health Department when it wrote that the "quality of life" was not in its purview.

A study of U.S bankruptcies tells a part of this scandalous story. Harvard Medical School's Steffie J. Woolhandler addressed a meeting of the Society of General Internal Medicine and said, "Among all debtors filing for bankruptcy, 55 percent...cited one or more medical causes...This is an incredibly profound indictment of healthcare financing in the United States."

Spending by the general population on its healthcare increases every year, similar to the growing governmental allocations per person for health that we mentioned earlier, now up to over $6,000 an individual. Healthcare expenses are now the third largest overall outlay in the U.S, surpassed only by the government and the retail industry. They are measured in the trillions and account for almost 15 percent of the total economy.

As getting sick is expensive for the individual in our society, so, too, is it costly to the taxpayers, the system, and the facilities. Sickness affects us all. Prevention would be a lot cheaper for everyone. And add to that the loss of a productive person's skills and labor to our diminishing "quality of life."

Our Dubious Honors

In a puzzling statement, as government think tanks keep crying out how we must control the healthcare dollar with all sorts of tightening-up rules and regulations and practices, the National Academy of Sciences stated that, rather, we must reward high-quality medical programs as a way of making better doctors and providing us with better facilities, from high tech ORs to chronic care nursing homes.

With health costs on the dole mounting, so are our national debts. A Herblock cartoon from 1986, in reporting that the U.S had just become the world's leading debtor nation, a place we have not since relinquished, sported the headline "We're Number One!" Tragically, we can make other similar dubious claims, as well.

What is the American paradox, as asked by political writer Ted Halstead in preparing us for yet another wild promise in a State of the Union address? That we are a nation with the most patents, Nobel laureates, and millionaires. But we are as well the world's leading industrialized country with the highest levels of poverty, homicide, and infant mortality.

We remain without a healthcare program that covers all our citizens. In presenting the data for this book to various publishing outlets and media moguls, I was told by more than one that healthcare and its need does not seem to be that important to people. I guess I should have answered by reminding them that they should think that over when they don't feel so well.

There is nothing more devastating than having poor health, but worse still is having a health deficiency that is undiagnosed, frightening, painful, and goes untreated for one reason or another. Nothing equals that feeling of powerlessness and frustration. Imagine, then, having such a feeling but with the added burden of never having hope or avenue of relief of any kind, much less a cure.

Philosophic comedian Sammy Levinson's favorite curse is that you should have enough wealth to have seven beautiful mansions, one for every day of the week, and in the garage of each mansion, you should have seven Rolls-Royce limousines, one for each day of the week, each with a different chauffeur, one for each day of the week. And every day, from each mansion, out of each garage, each of the different chauffeurs should take you in a different Rolls-Royce limo to a different doctor, and not one of them is able to tell you what is wrong with you. ♦

CHAPTER 3

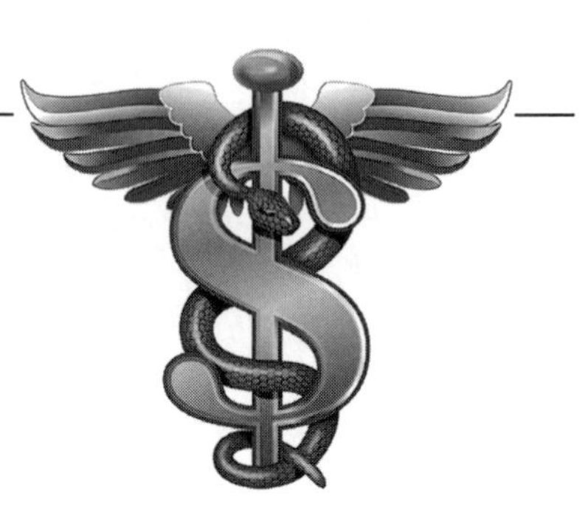

Doctors Are Developed, Not Erupted—The Art of Medicine

Just a few years ago, one of the country's eminent clinicians, a medical school department chairman from the "old school," published in a leading medical journal an article titled "The Modern Day Resident in Obstetrics and Gynecology—A Marvel in Electronic Technology." It was his way of lamenting to his colleagues that we indeed may have over-computerized and hi-tech-designed our doctors-in-training. In the ebbing years of his teaching career, he had seen that hands-on, eyes-on, ears-on, nose-on, tongue-on approach to patient care had been replaced in good part by the LED blips of an electronic monitor, the sonar waves of an ultrasound device, and the dots and dashes of a software DVD inside a computerized, anodized metal box.

The physician-in-training who someday will be administering to a live human being may, on that day, be sitting at a nursing station down the hall while his patient is at the other end of the corridor, perhaps even on another floor in the hospital, in another city, or, wait, in another country.

In this world of modern medicine, major surgical procedures are carried out by stainless steel robots under the electronic guidance of a surgeon who is perhaps perched in a cubicle sometimes thousands of miles away. The robots' hands are probes, look-alikes mimicking a prosthesis, projections that wield instruments and surgical devices that are manipulated by the human surgeon from that kind of distance. Commonplace? Of course not. Not yet, anyway.

But such an illustration does point out what may be in store for us. For better or for worse, this may be a signal that the human touch has been relegated to a secondary role, or at least has a shared role of some sort with the modern world of computer technology, a world which is now a half-century old and has already provided us with wonders beyond our imaginations. I am sure that people sat back and wondered what the wheel would bring them, or what electricity, the telephone, and television harkened. They all brought us further along on a journey into a never-never land.

The computer is a machine that only has the power and ability to say "yes" or "no," but can, by saying it fast enough, create a mathematics beyond our dreams. A building model that can mimic the human animal. And with an accuracy that is sometimes scary.

Modern Technology

The good news is that this technology can save lives. The question remains—is something new automatically better? Has technology made better doctors and better medicine? All by itself? Or when applied at the right time and in the right quantity?

One medical author described a visit to a twenty-first-century labor and delivery suite in a large California coast city medical center. He peered inside, where upwards of thirty newborns were spending their first few days of life, and he felt he was in a NASA tracking station in Houston. The maze of equipment, machinery, glowing monitors, and all sizes of screens tracking the welfares of the neonates was head-spinning. It took him a second to locate the patient-babies. They were indeed there, buried under all that equipment. And while there were a zillion nurses and aides flittering about, there was also that battery of physicians and technician specialists at some outside desk, following the blips and LED numbers on a screen, just as though they were watching their patients. Which they were. Or, at least what was to them the equivalent of their patients. Did that medical center boast of better demographics than others less "fortunate" to have such equipment? No. They all came out even. It seemed to depend on something else.

What, then, does it take to make a better baby? A more healthy newborn? A sturdier and more robust kid? The answer is clear: the proper combination of technology, science, and intimate patient care. I was trained as a medical student on my first tour of duty in pediatrics by a wise old gent, standing only five foot four and sporting 250 pounds of girth, with a lavish, Gildersleeve-type mustache, who taught that before we were ever to prescribe a medication for our pediatric patient of any size or type, we had to take a drop of it on our finger and touch it to the tip of our tongues. That way, we would always know its taste and consistency. We were never to give a baby something we hadn't sampled ourselves. It was the start of making us humble.

The Five Senses

The man given credit as the proverbial "father of medicine," the Greek scholar Hippocrates, would have been mighty proud of my first pediatric professor. He followed the tenets of Hippocrates, by all lore and recounts, and was indeed a hands-on physician. And all the other "ons." His medical students, steeped in that tradition, were taught to use their given senses in treating their patients. His students were never permitted to prescribe a medication for a child before first sampling it by dipping a cotton-tipped applicator and touching it to the tip of the tongue. He wanted the student doctors to experience what the patient would. This was a lesson in empathy they never would forget.

I recall walking down the hospital corridor one afternoon with my surgical instructor taking a call from a postoperative patient who had complained of severe pain. As we approached the patient's room, my instructor turned to me and said, "He has a wound abscess." Puzzled, I awaited to see if his prognostication was valid, secretly hoping it wasn't, thus returning the lesson of humility. It was.

"How were you so sure?" I asked. He pointed to the tip of his nose, took a short sniff, and said he smelled it twenty feet away. I had my first lesson in the value of the pheromone, that biochemical substance secreted by every animal that stimulates an olfactory, physiological, and behavioral response to any individual of the same species. Though not as highly developed in the human as in other lower animals that use them to identify an enemy or to attract mates, it is there just the same. The art of special odor detection and interpretation of human purulence, and with particular traits depending on where they secrete from, was never forgotten. Fecal smell is unlike oral odor, and so forth. Since then, I have never walked toward a patient in need without starting that short sniff exercise as I approach her bedside. I have even learned to lift the covers and take a deep breath. ♦

The computer can only say "yes" or "no." It cannot see, hear, smell, taste, or touch. Only the living animal can do such things. Investigative determinations or instinctual findings elucidated by communication and consult among physicians, nurses, and lab technicians result in better patient care. When indications are better communicated, there are better cures. That is why medicine has earned the added descriptor as an "art" rather than a "science."

A career in medicine is one that is essentially universal. You pay your dues and you go through your paces on a defined linear route to advancement. All across the globe, medical school training is remarkably similar. Physicians are not surprised, therefore, when we meet another from among our ranks, from some distant place, who talks the same "language." In fact, it has been shown many times over that the better cure rates and progresses in dealing with pathology are much improved when treatment of an ailment has benefited from a universal discourse and communication.

In the field of gynecology, for example, one of the greatest accomplishments over the past scores of years has been the cure and survival rate of what was once a most deadly disease—cancer of the female cervix. But while radiology, surgery, chemo, and most of all, the Papanicolaou smear (for prevention and early detection, which meant a cure) came into being, a key to successfully fighting the disease has been the international classification that has allowed for worldwide exchange. This has enabled the entire world's medical community to understand and translate one oncologist's treatment to another's, and women the world over have been rewarded by that continuity of care. Fewer got lost in the shuffle. And more survive.

Computers cannot do such things. A machine that says only "yes" or "no" just doesn't cut it. People should take care of people.

The Continuity of Care

A story from the Cuban socialist revolution that changed the entire economic and social structure of that island nation is another vivid case in point.

Before 1959, during the Batista regime that had kept Cuba as a colonial property of the Western world and its corporate conglomerates, the Cuban people were in dire medical straits. In 1958, for example, one out of every five Cubano newborns (read: the poor) died within the first twenty-eight days of life from what we now know is coliform diarrhea, a syndrome contracted from poor sanitation and lack of potable water. By 1972, that cause of morbidity and mortality had just about been eliminated through a massive construction blueprint for modern sewer and sanitation plants, and preventive care.

As a part of Cuba's newly created medical system, under which medical training centers were built and serviced by crops of trained healthcare professionals, the mass numbers of Cubans who had never even seen the insides of a clinic or doctor's office for any sort of care were suddenly and happily exposed to clinics. Called polyclinics to indicate the ubiquitousness of their services, they existed in ghetto neighborhoods as well in the hinterlands of the island.

Generalists and all types of family practitioners held regular office hours, served their communities, and sent the patients to the major urban medical centers for specialized care, as the specialties became available over the years of the post-revolutionary government.

But a strange thing happened that hadn't been predicted. Well into the new polyclinic system, the patient population became dissatisfied, despite their sudden access to care and cures they never experienced or thought ever to be possible. The women, for example, complained that during their pregnancies, after being followed by a family doctor whom they had come to know and trust, who was a part of their neighborhood and even a part of the family, so to speak, they were, once in labor at the end of their gestations, sent off to the lying-in hospital and put under the care of obstetrically trained specialists. That they delivered fine, healthy newborns somehow still left them with feelings of deprivation.

Investigations and surveys finally revealed the problem. What was missing was a continuity of care. The patient had become accustomed to her regular doctor and felt rejected and abandoned when she was suddenly thrust into the care of another doctor, however capable, at that time of acute need.

Many other patients felt the same. Men who went through various gyrations with their family physicians for their cardiac or other chronic care were also sent off to specialty hospitals whenever hospitalization was called for, and that continuity was broken. Yes, the supervision of a specialist was needed, to be sure, but the friendly face of that neighborhood *doctoro* was missing.

Changes were made. Despite a rather successful medical delivery system that was easily and obviously light years ahead of what the poor had had in the Cuba before the revolution, this need had to be addressed. The family polyclinic doctor became obligated to accompany the patient to the hospital to help in the delivery of his/her parturient.

The doctor also retained control of the man who went off for intrahospital care for his cardiac condition or gall bladder surgery or whatever, made daily bedside visits, and actively participated in the patient's care.

That all made sense to the Western medical community, which was closely following the progress of the Cuban system. One of the stark differences in U.S. care for the private and clinic group of patients had always been a realization of that lack of continuity, something that, under the U.S. system, seemingly could not be corrected. The hospital clinic patients here, under a for-profit system, automatically became teaching cases for the residents and student doctors, and this created a change in the definitions of both patient and doctor.

There have been some hospitals and residency training programs that have recognized this failing and have tried, often in vain, to adjust. Some have adopted what is called a vertical team system, where a staff attending heads a group of several others at all levels of experience, from chief resident to the first year, that is responsible for a complement of patients. Someone on the vertical team must always be on call to address patient needs and care. That way, the patients always understand and accept the same group that comes to be known as their doctor(s). This seemed to correct some of that loss of continued care, but not all, since staff assignments change or a semester of training ends, and when others are put in charge, the patients lose their doctors forever. But at least it was a start and an acknowledgement of the problem at hand.

The long odyssey that takes a budding medical student through the years of medical education has not changed that much in the centuries since Hippocrates. Yes, it has become more and more specialized, but training programs and so-called fellowships have still had to accept the unchanged uniformity in instruction that has defined the modern era. The medical didactic authorities have delineated a more or less critical minimum for training, below which no physician can be certified for practice, obviously for the protection of the patient.

The theory of continuity of care as an aspect of patient management is also behind the laws that require national citizenship in order to practice medicine. This curtails the use of transient doctors and also serves as a reminder that clinicians are a type of servant of their patients. To provide optimal healing, doctors must identify with their patients' social lifestyles, family values, and mores. It is like applying a broad, cotton-wrapped applicator to the tip of your tongue to sample a patient's lifestyle, home environment, and habits. Using such insights to heal is truly applying the Hippocratic model of medicine as an art, not a science.

The Premedical Prep

The premed years have their value as well in cementing the "art" side of medicine. The founding fathers (not too many mothers back then) wisely decided that physicians must have some sort of background in the arts, as well as the sciences. Thus, to physics, biology, math, and organic chemistry were added at least a smattering in English grammar and some exposure to a foreign language. Medical school admission committees seek out the broadest possible eventual student. Courses in any of the arts, from music to literature, as part of their premedical training, weighed heavily in the candidates' favor. Medical schools like well-rounded prospects.

Medical schools also like it when those students graduate. In fact, one of the medical school rating agencies in the world of academia looks to the percentage of those students who graduate four years later based on the number that started out. A 100 precent graduation record is sought. Certainly, in all U.S. medical schools working in our educational system, a student drop-out after the start of the third year due to scholastic failure is most unusual. Schools make very special efforts to keep their students moving forward. Tutors, extra classes, and even professorial counseling are available when a student falters.

There are many top flight schools that announce to the first-year class on opening day that "There are 'X' number of students starting, and there will be 'X' students graduating." This gives a clear and concise message that academic wavering is seriously frowned upon.

The first half of a standard four-year program is spent on the preclinical subjects. Anatomy, physiology, and histology, the microscopic study of the body's cells, make the core of the first year curriculum.

The sophomores study pathology, biochemistry, and pharmacology, all as a segue to the upcoming third and fourth clinical years. Added to this are introduction courses to basic psychiatry, clinical disease syndromes, and now, preliminary training in the world of medical computer technology, the wave of the future.

The candidate is thus prepared to enter his/her (about evenly divided now) two last clinical years. These are divided almost evenly in the classrooms covering surgery, pediatrics, advanced psychiatry, obstetrics and gynecology, and general internal medicine. Finally come more advanced medicine and some of the subspecialties, such as radiology, oncology, laboratory pathology, and more computer technology.

It was once thought that these four years, plus a so-called required fifth year known as an internship, when the students spend all their time in a hospital setting under guided actual patient care, was preparation enough to move forward. It was assumed then that at that point, the embryonic doctor is sufficiently schooled to present for a set of written and practical oral board exams, either of the type that is national and universal in scope and accepted by every state in the United States, or a different exam that allows for some amount of reciprocity within the fifty states. That has now changed.

Today, the internship has more or less been relegated to the history books. Specialization is so commonplace that a single one-year, hospital-based experience is deemed insufficient and inadequate. The world of medicine has become so complex and technical that the training period allotted in the old model has become too brief. As more and more knowledge of the human body and mind is exposed, more and more time is needed to grasp its workings. Factor into that the constantly growing technology, and still more training is needed.

There are those medical centers of learning that are gradually recognizing that the psychological aspects of the human being must be explored for physicians to better and fully understand their patients. As a case in point, psychiatry, as the study of human behavior, is working its way into an earlier part of the medical school agenda. This specialty, which used to be offered in the third or fourth year, has now been put into the first year of the core curriculum. Social concepts such as racism, nationalism, and sexism are becoming part of the medical school disciplines.

The Gender Gap

There is as well the growth brought about by increasing numbers of women to the field as they are becoming more and more a part of the medical community. Although behind other developed nations, where medical and dental schools are inundated with female candidates, the U.S. is shifting in certain specialties that are becoming more attractive to women. Pediatrics, internal medicine, obstetrics and gynecology, and the non-clinical specialties such as radiology, pathology, pharmacology, and hematology first attracted the female medical student. But urology, orthopedics, and general surgery are seeing the changes as more women are joining their ranks. Indeed, it is no longer unusual to have clinical programs that in the past were strictly male, open now to all comers.

As an intern in internal medicine back in the early '60s, I recall being assigned to one of our attendings, Dr. Bernard Samuels. He was a man of mid-sixties with a robust practice and a fine reputation as a clinician and, more importantly for me, a teacher. Being assigned to his service was a privilege and a treat. My job description included getting the regular, almost daily, list of Dr. Samuels' hospital admissions. I was to visit the patients, welcome them to the hospital, do an initial history and physical, and then await Dr Samuels for our late afternoon teaching rounds.

On one occasion, I started my round with Albert Gustufson, a man of seventy-one, who more or less looked his stated age. A glance at the chart told the sad story. Al Gustufson was a widower of several years, his children and grandchildren devoted but no longer living in the area. He had been a chain smoker off and on, a moderate social drinker, and only a gall bladder removal at age fifty and a partial pulmonary resection surgery four years prior were significant. A cough and chest cramps some years ago brought him to Dr. Samuels and the diagnosis of lung cancer was confirmed. It had been hoped that the resection would do the trick. No such luck.

The cancer had at first spread locally and the patient needed more help. Al had been in and out of the hospital under the care of Dr. Samuels and appeared stabilized. But the cough became more persistent and no longer responded to Dr. Samuels' palliation. It was time for some more in-depth evaluation and intense treatment.

Patient Gustufson was tall and lanky and was sitting with his legs draped over an ottoman over in the corner of his private room, listening and watching attentively to the 5 o'clock news. He had been through this drill before. He was waiting for my visit, chat, and exam. His snow-white hair and one-day beard growth surrounded a long face, pursed lips. He had a high-pitched, friendly, crackly voice. We became friends in no time. A medium-sized ashtray with a beanbag base already had two small butts, and he snuffed the one he was dragging on as soon as I approached. The no-smoking rule that has become strictly enforced and universal in all U.S. hospitals and so many other public buildings was not yet in effect. It was a few years away.

Al pointed his index finger to my lower back and scrunched up his face and eyes as he described the aches that just weren't relieved by anything he knew to do. He obviously was assuming that Dr. Samuels and I were going to have the magic bullet. I must have seemed a little puzzled, and we made some small talk while waiting for Dr. Samuels to appear. I felt congenial enough to first name the patient. "Al," I started off, "I got to get you to break that damn smoking habit. We got to get you out of trouble, and that is a good way to start. I don't have to tell you that your young grandchildren might look at you as a role model. I bet you want to teach them good and safe habits."

Al Gustufson looked at me, nodded, and, more meaningfully, squashed the smoldering cigarette into the ashtray. "Good advice," he muttered.

Dr. Samuels arrived. They made the appropriate small talk, and Mr. Gustufson wasted no time. "Doc," he was addressing his physician, "this young whippersnapper of a doctor did for me in ten minutes what you have been badgering me about for years. No more smokes for me. No, sir. I am quitting as of this moment. Got to get myself better for my kids."

Bernie Samuels smiled, took the chart out of my hands, and leafed through a few pages. He looked up, handed me the all bent up aluminum clipboard, and turned to his patient. "Al," he said very calmly but with deliberation, "the young doctor is right, of course. But he was not aware of some of the latest lab studies we did on you. The numbers are different. No problem with your smoking anymore. Your situation is stable enough for you to puff away. Enjoy."

Gustufson reached for the open pack on the nightstand, shook out the last one, and flicked his well-worn stainless steel lighter and lit up. "OK, Doctor Samuels, you are the boss." The two exchanged a few more comments about what was being planned in the way of testing the following day and how long he would have to stay this time around. They shook hands, and we went out the door together. I waved my hand to all with a motion that was a kind of an apology for being second-guessed, and we both parted with a smile.

Out in the corridor, heading to our next patient call, Dr. Samuels turned to me and gave me my first pearl of the day. Knowing his reputation, there were many more yet to come. "Sloan," he said, "Al Gustufson has been smoking for the past sixty-five years. Almost two packs a day. I diagnosed his squamous cell about three years ago. First came the resection, then chemo trials, and a few other things. I will give you the complete run down." He handed me a photocopy of his office file sheet with the panorama of Gustufson's history and visits.

"Al is not going to make it," he went on. "He may leave the hospital this time, but maybe not. I just saw his latest chest plates, and he is loaded. Those backaches are mets that weren't there last week. They go from C4 to S3." That was Dr. Samuels' way of anatomically describing the metastases from the fourth cervical spinal notch way down to the third sacral. That was just about the whole spine.

I was not yet totally aware of what was coming. "So we aren't going to do much more for him than some back rubs, now lots of aspirin, and eventually, lots more of other analgesics. The big guns. You know what I mean. He is going to go downhill over the next couple of weeks or so, and we will make him as comfortable as possible until we lose him. I already told his sister. She said she will call his son if he can be located. They haven't been in touch for years. Maybe the guy is dead. Don't know."

I was beginning to get the gruesome picture. "Al Gustufson is about to become another cigarette statistic. It makes no sense to deny him what little pleasure he has left." I gave an understanding double blink. ♦

Medical Pearls Learned

The tragedy of an Al Gustufson would be repeated again and again, many, many times before my internship and residency years were over. They would wear different faces and have different histories. But they would all be human dramas. They were the things that could only be taught and learned by a devoted and experienced clinician who was willing to spend the time it took to impart these nuggets to a willing, eager, and attentive student.

These were the medical pearls not picked up from a computer blip or a set of LED numbers. Nor could they ever become a part of the chart legends, X-ray plates, or laboratory columns. Eventually, that paper chart and the metal clipboard were going to be replaced, as they are as we speak, by a set of software discs. There will no longer be that pile of progress records that could be leafed through by the doctors on rounds so that they could look back and reflect on what was handwritten and interpreted as part of the complexity of that human drama, unfolding during the course of a patient's illness. Instead, there would be a laptop or desktop, or even more streamlined, a Blackberry that reveals data one screen at a time, as the house staff or attendings push buttons and roll levers in order to discern the whole picture. Like that professor wrote—the modern day medical staffer is a wonder in computer wizardry.

Do you think for a minute that all this technology that paves the road with good intentions on the way to hell is unrelated to what is happening in a profit-driven healthcare system? Don't believe that, not for one moment.

As nations around the world devote more of their time and resources to medical technology, the people who do not get better fast enough and often enough are still not going to get better fast enough or often enough. The technocrats that are softwaring medical care are putting their eggs in one basket. The haves are getting what is being construed as some form of medical progress, allowing always that better and better communication can improve healthcare delivery. Remember what has happened to cervical cancer in women this past half-century since the advent of the PAP smear and the international exchange of that data.

But advanced computer technology in offices, hospitals, nursing stations, and clinics, and all that that means, has no value in places where there are no offices, hospitals, nursing stations, and clinics, and moreover, where there are no trained people to use them. That is all more for the haves and less for the have nots.

As unlimited as we think our resources are, and they are vast, people will be spending more and more of their incomes on living longer and living better. Up to a point. There comes a time when the return starts to diminish. That is when it is time to stop and think what we are doing on that home front.

U.S. healthcare costs have already passed the 15 percent mark of our gross national income levels, and that is ever climbing this very moment. Other nations in the developed world that have some semblance of government-sponsored healthcare for their people are also seeing similar increases in their own backyards. Do not ask me why, but those nations take it as some form of accomplishment to ape what the USA is doing on that absurd level. They never seem to take into account that there are those 80 million plus Americans who have inadequate healthcare coverage or none at all.

Childbirth Paves the Way

In the world of obstetrics, the Lamaze natural childbirth movement started gaining real momentum in the 1960s. Ferdinand Lamaze was a Frenchman who did much of his research and clinical trials with natural childbirth in his native France, with his *accouchement sans douleur,* and later on in Moscow. Yet, the United States, being what it is at the forefront of so many movements, soon became the center of his teaching and work. The American Lamaze schools took over and led the way for the world to copy.

When computerized and machine-monitored labor and delivery entered into the U.S. obstetrical scene a couple of decades later, newfangled instant epidurals came into vogue. Women went into labor and were immediately hooked up to those NASA-like gadgets, wrapped in belts, monitors, electrodes, and electronic clips that were essentially measuring every facet of fetal and maternal functioning. Like I said, the doctor and nurse could and did sit out at a weigh station in front of a maze of electronic screens and gadgetry, watching the course of labor. Red warning lights blinked if the numbers did not act according to a given norm.

Those who were from the old school that used a medical student's ear and hands as a monitor of fetal and maternal progress and their own ears and eyes as guides of labor's course insisted that back in the old countries, France and Russia, a more human approach was still being applied to the *accouchement* and added a reminder that perinatal and maternal mortality and morbidity statistics were no worse than our own.

It was earlier on in my teaching excursions to Cuba in the mid-seventies as that island nation was building up its doctor population. I was an annual guest lecturer in obstetrics, learning as much about Third World labor and delivery as I taught.

In one session, I had finished my work and rounds through the ward and labor room and noticed the frenzy such places have when a few more women in labor come in than are anticipated. Obstetrics is not exactly a predictable workload or science. Over the espresso pot during a break in the action, I chatted with the director of the lying-in unit, Doctoro Pedro Valdez Vivo, a distinguished clinician before the revolution. We spoke of my suggestion that for my next visit during the coming year I might include teaching aids for the implementation of the Lamaze method of natural childbirth and even the use of trained midwives that were coming into vogue in many areas in the U.S. This was credited with helping relieve the busy OBS clinicians of the burden of tending to the normal deliveries that made up the vast bulk of any patient load. My comments were immediately greeted with a shake of the head.

"That is not for us, at least not yet, and maybe never," Doctoro Valdez Vivo said. "Our men folks are not used to such involvement. Baby delivery is woman's work. Men tend to the fields and the workplace. At least for now. Besides, your so-called natural childbirth with the glamour of modern labor and delivery suites and numerous personnel and well-equipped facilities is a luxury for the wealthy and comfortable, not the poor and needy. Your underprivileged in the States must also have a mindset that keeps them in the workplace to prepare for their impending new families. Haves and have nots are no different the world over. Your Americano Lamaze methods are a treat for the women who can afford

the pleasure of private nurses, labor coaches, and preparation classes. Here, we have to worry about delivering healthy babies, something our people are not yet used to." Pedro Valdez Vivo smiled, as he knew I understood his words and thoughts.

He went on. "Midwives? That is something else again, although not for us. That is political and emotional, all in one." Professor Valdez Vivo filled his demitasse-sized cup with dark coffee and heaps of sugar.

"During the struggle to implement the revolution, it was Commandante Fidel Castro and his comrades who sought support and help for the revolutionary process. He reminded the peasants that at one time, the poor people of Cuba used local huts and even barnyard hay piles as delivery rooms, and all without doctors or even nurses or knowledgeable people in case there were troubles. Many babies died in childbirth. The Commandante swore to his people that if they helped him win the struggle, we would have hospitals and doctors and trained and schooled obstetricians who would have all women give birth to their newborns in the security of a hospital setting with them on hand. Anything else now would be looked upon as a betrayal of that promise."

I stood back and reached for another cup of cool water. Labor and delivery suites then had no air conditioning. I had just gotten a lesson in obstetrics never taught in my stateside hospital center—the human side of medicine. An art, not a science. ♦

Then there was that rude awakening. Good ol' American know-how was being exported. They wanted to be like us, so the fetal monitors and computers and screens slowly made their way into European L&D's. Many an *accouchement sans douleur* has now become *accouchement avec l'ordinator*, or *le computer*, in French-English parlance.

Keeping Up

It is evident that Americans, Japanese, and Europeans are spending more of their incomes on their health, if only to keep up with the costs of the ever growing and newly introduced technology. Yes, because of the greater administrative costs associated with constantly growing technology that are uniquely American, profit margins rise sharply. The cost of healthcare rises. And strides in technology are certainly more prominent in the U.S. than their Second World counterparts with their healthcare programs.

Heart bypass surgery is performed several times more often per capita in the U.S. than in the industrialized nations of Western Europe, the G-7 countries, or in Canada with their federally sponsored healthcare. Are French and Canadian hearts healthier than ours? Could that be? To the tune of seven or more times? Of course not. Indications for surgery are quite different among the three, obviously reserved for the more extreme cases in Europe and Canada.

Important to note, of course, is that those same demographics clearly indicate that the Canadian and French people do not suffer with any greater cardiac morbidity than we do, and our cardiac mortality stats are essentially the same.

It is clear: Those nations that have federal healthcare plans that minimize the profits of the medical industry have equal success and results. U5MR's are about equal. And they have less expensive technology, to boot.

It was the first week in July, traditionally when new house staffs have come on board at the teaching hospitals. Medical students that would not have been trusted with a sick puppy dog the day before just had a night's sleep on June 30 and woke up the next morning on July first as licensed physicians, with all of the legal and moral responsibility that goes with it. Overnight, they got that stamp of approval.

On morning rounds in a medical ward, the chief resident had his starched-uniformed team standing at attention as the teaching attending staff joined in promptly at the designated hour. Rounds always started on time.

The group went from bedside to bedside, each case presented by one of the house officers, and, after a few sage comments by the attending doctors, the case was opened for questions and discussion. The sessions were usually lively and friendly.

In Ward Room 22A, they came to the bedside of a fiftyish appearing male, in no apparent acute distress. The professor-doctor in charge and the rest of the group heard the chief resident's summary history as they had every day for the past two weeks. The patient's case was a conundrum. There had been no confirmed diagnosis, and the treatment so far was symptomatic and palliative.

In the rear of the crowd at bedside stood a newcomer, the first-year resident in the group, one of those who had walked down the aisle at his own medical school graduation in June and had now joined the crew.

At the first break in the action, after some perfunctory exchanges among the staff, the youngster of the crowd raised his hand to speak. After a nod of recognition, he asked, "How about agnogenic myeloid metaplasia?" This was greeted with a stark moment of silence. The pathology mentioned was as esoteric a one you could find, being an oddball blood dyscrasia of a rather serious nature and likely not seen in the combined medical careers of all present. It was still in the medical textbooks as an existing syndrome and although relegated primarily to those pages, there were cases that once in a while popped up in the world.

"Has AMM been screened?" asked the chief officer. "Okay, let's run it through the lab," he said with a tone of dismissal rather than serious contemplation.

A few days later, the group collected themselves again for their morning rounds. When they reached 22A's bedside, the chief resident sheepishly looked up from his clipboard and announced to the staff that indeed the AMM test was returned as positive, and treatment was underway.

The head attending muttered a few choice words to his colleagues and looked up at the new junior resident. "Nice diagnosis and interesting evaluation. Tell us, what in the patient and his record made you think of AMM?" This could obviously be a babe-in-the-woods teaching point that was worth making.

"Oh," replied the lad, "I had read about it a few weeks ago in preparing for my board exams and figured that I would just say it for every case that had gone undiagnosed, and I might get lucky and be right-on eventually." The staff moved on without comment. ♦

Medicine is an art, not a science.

What was passed on by Dr. Samuels and the exchanges at bedside 22A are daily occurrences. Many times daily. Nuances are transferred by eye contact, hints, casual conversation, and a nod of the head. It has been said that you can tell the level of training and sophistication of a physician by the amount of time she/he takes to turn over a patient to a colleague or covering doctor.

When you are a medical student, just getting your proverbial feet wet in medicine, and you are about to leave for the weekend, it takes about two hours to describe and outline your set of, say, twenty patients in your charge. When you are a second-year resident, that same chore needs about half that time. By your final year as chief resident, it take sabout twenty minutes, and after a few years around the block, with the experience of a practicing clinician, turning over a whole practice for the weekend or vacation would take about ten minutes. Why? Because with more experience comes more confidence and the ability to filter the patients' problems and histories down to a bare—but vital and sufficient—minimum.

Appropriately named, Professor Willie Dock, M.D. was my third-year medical school preceptor. I was one of six students who lucked out and drew his name. Doctor Dock was a wiry 135 pounds soaking wet and stood at about five foot six with a sharp voice that matched his morphology. His office in the Department of Medicine was on the eighth floor of the hospital, and he almost never saw the inside of an elevator. He used the stairwell twice a day, five days a week. Not recommended. Weekends were for his bicycle.

As a widower, his only vacations were two weeks at the famous Kempner Institute at Duke University in North Carolina, where he lived on rice (white, no less) and exercises planned to keep him alive till one hundred. He almost made it.

It was always considered a mark of accomplishment as a medical student of the house officer if you were able to impress Willie Dock. His nod in your direction was like brewing that perfect cup of coffee for Alexa Gente. So when I was assigned to present a case on Monday morning grand rounds, I immediately put everything else aside to spend the weekend getting ready for my fifteen minutes of fame. I made a patient bedside visit on Saturday, stopped in at the chemistry and hematology labs and radiology to confirm the chart reports, and spent a couple of hours in the school library to be sure I was up on the latest literature. I couldn't have felt more confident.

The bewitching hour arrived, and the whole group of about twenty-five assembled on the ward. No one missed a Doctor Dock teaching rounds. The chief resident motioned for the first case, and I was on. I gave what I thought was a brilliant patient history with his admitting complaints, the resident and attending physical exam findings, all the lab data, and the differential diagnoses. I anticipated Doctor Dock's nod of approval.

"How well did he sleep last night?" was the opening question. I hesitated, not exactly sure of the answer. "Any change in his pain pattern?" came next. I answered in a general way, not wanting to get tripped up with any misinformation. "Did he void okay? How about his bowel movement? Did he have any problems on the weekend?" I stood in silence. Doctor Dock wasn't done. Finally, he asked," What did your patient eat yesterday for dinner, Sloan? Did he enjoy it?" I was flabbergasted, not being absolutely sure of a single answer.

Doctor Dock waited for a brief moment in a deafen silence and then took the floor. I felt relieved if only because at least all eyes switched from me to the professor.

"It is all well and good to be up on your patient's history, what brought him here in the first place, and all that chart data. Very important. But do not forget for one moment that what you have in front of you in that bed is a human being, and in trouble. How much we don't know yet. His behavior, like anyone's, is unpredictable. How be slept, BM'd, pee-peed, his aches and pains, and his appetite will not be found on any lab print out, X-ray plate, or EKG strip. Not till it's too late, maybe. First ask, listen to his answers, and you will hear how this human being is faring. Then you will digest all of that, add in the chart numbers, and you might just come up with a diagnosis and management. Rembrandt was an artist. So are you."

A valuable lesson never forgotten. From that moment on, I have never made a patient visit without taking along my easel, palette, and brush.

At our last session of the semester, ready to enter our fourth and final year, Doctor Willie Dock had each of his students promise that if we were ever to come across him in the street in need of dire medical help during July or August after that fateful first June 30, we were to keep on walking, save perhaps to make sure his feet and socks were clean before he went to a hospital. He would never want to be put into the hands of a new-born physician during those first sixty days.

We needed that much time to realize the art in medicine. Until we did, he would prefer to be left to his own devices. ♦

A Little Bit of Both

There is an association between that art of medicine and what has happened to the technology now involved and what priority we put on it. That medical center nursery in California that looks like a NASA control center can boast of no better results than the centers with less paraphernalia but with caring, well trained, and up-to-date clinicians.

Why? Because high falutin' technology, although it certainly has its place in modern medicine, has as well been over-sold to an unsuspecting public as the answer to many of medicine's failings. Hi-tech medicine is related directly to the economics of the industry, and as long as medical care is looked upon as a privilege with a profit motive, everything else involved will as well—such as malpractice insurance, the pharmaceuticals, hospital supplies, hi-tech equipment, and instrumentation. Why not? As with any business, if the bottom line is the financial bottom line, then everyone involved has that right to improve theirs. Makes sense.

But it then becomes a question of priority. What is the medical industry there for? I repeat. Bottom line or patient care?

The whole world can and would benefit from the advances in health technology, albeit driven by the allure of the profits that can be made. Those developed nations that have their semblances of "socialized" forms of healthcare delivery but are now inching toward the U.S. model of hi-tech may be in for quite a surprise as their healthcare costs mount.

Already, the governments of Canada and Great Britain are feeling the sting of hi-tech costs: funding for their federal programs is getting tighter and tighter. Complaints are being heard about the delays in offered services. As market forces dictate the quality and quantity of the services available, and those funds get reduced, the pinch in the care for the people grows. Just like here at home in the USA, as Ten Downing Street spends too much in Baghdad and the Falkland (Malvenas) Island campaign, it spends less on national health services. The people are bound to suffer. That is exactly what is happening.

Doctors-in-training are finding themselves more involved in the computer wizardry of their hospitals and schools as the answer to improving healthcare delivery. Sharp-talking salespeople with their own axes to grind are hard selling hospital administrators that the hi-tech direction is the way to go as a means of showing their collective devotion to patient care. Over these upcoming decades, modern societies will be debating the value of hi-tech versus hands-on medicine.

Hospitals are boasting that they are becoming "paperless." That the clipboard and the manila folder that hold the patients' histories and progress notes are becoming history themselves, and patient records are now only viewed on that monitor screen. The trade off is grey. There must be a way to coordinate the art of medicine and allow for that Norman Rockwell image while incorporating the best of what twenty-first-century medicine has to offer.

Many at medical board meetings and conferences are asking the question—the electronic medical record—is it for us?

The MS-DOS (Microsoft Disk Operating System) has been around for over a score of years, but has been understood by only the very literate, usually those doctors with children of primary school age in the household who were becoming computer-skilled and teaching the rest of the family. Even then, however, physicians were using it as a toy or hobby, playing solitaire and blackjack as much as anything. In the next several years, after some of the house and nursing staffs took the required courses run by outside computer salespeople at the hospitals, the docs, playing dumb and claiming "you can't teach an old dog new tricks," had to wait out at the nursing station to get someone to bring up the proper screen and get lab data and other patient results. That welcome finally wore thin.

"Get with the program—or else," was the warning. The attending staff, no matter how senior, soon came to realize that the art of medicine included going electronic. One excuse offered was that there were not enough years left to learn new tricks. But even for them, it just became more practical to learn how to punch the right buttons and weave around the mouse rather than sit about and wait for help.

The twenty-first century is leaving doctors no other choice. They are reluctantly joining the game. There is no guess as to how long it will take to complete the turnover. The old dogs will be learning new tricks.

Some years ago, one member from a northeastern state rose to introduce a bill. He declared that it was time for the USA to go metric on the floor of the U.S. Senate. That we were the only nation left in the world that persisted in using the English system and that our manufacturers were having the added expense of making almost two separate products, one with the English system for domestic sales, and the other with metric gauges for overseas shipment. And since we were odd man out, it was time to play catch up.

While the Senate pondered a bit, most of the argument making good sense, a senator from a midwestern state took the floor. Yes, he said, that was all true, but there was a major drawback. He reminded his colleagues that his state and most others had the older citizens to consider, those who were long out of school and had no chance to learn anew. He described major confusion and disarray. The senior citizens would be at a great disadvantage, perhaps beyond repair.

His colleague hesitated and said, yes, that was so true and would be unfair. But since the change he suggested was needed, when could the change be made?

Simple, said the other legislator. When all the old people are dead. ♦

Medicine Taking Its Place in the Modern World

Medicine as an industry is already now our third biggest commodity. Only the government and retailing have greater numbers. This was not always true. The healthcare dollar costs are rising rapidly, faster than the others. Medical schools, even state supported and subsidized, have tuitions that are beyond reach for most Americans. Without some form of scholarship, many well-qualified candidates are denied only because they cannot possibly afford the tariff. And this when we are in need of doctors.

The awkward distribution of physicians in any society has always been a bone of contention. At the same time UNICEF and the other UN health arms were concocting the U5MR and other demographics for study, they also were determining the optimum patient:doctor ratio as a mark of the healthcare of any given nation. It was thus decided that the ideal for any country would be 180:1, or one doctor per 180 population. That is a goal that has been quite elusive for most countries in the world. Only Israel and Cuba have managed to succeed so far.

The countries of the G-7, the developed world of Western Europe and some of the east, have ratios that can be considered near adequate. Italy, Belgium, France, and a few more hover around the 220 mark; on the other end of the scale are the sub-Saharan nations in Africa with one doctor often per 20,000 or more people. Other nations in the Third World, even those in South America, are at about 1,000:1, or more. The U.S. ranks about where expected, given the two-tier system and lack of that universal program and also considering that physicians are free to practice where they please and without any incumbencies or obligations for service.

Thus, America's 320:1 ratio is somewhat distorted. In some areas, like in major urban centers and the affluent neighborhoods, the number could go as low as 40:1, but in the rural South may rise as high as 1,500:1.

Certainly, as part of any future national healthcare plan, those discrepancies would have to be evened out to better serve all communities. When put into action, any such plan would call for obligatory service by appropriate medical school graduates to fill those voids.

Government intervention into the careers of doctors on some fair and equal basis must be accepted. Just as more medical personnel are needed, their placement around the country plays a large role in updating and optimizing the healthcare of the nation. Too, the different specialties must be well and fairly distributed so as to keep people's needs in mind. As the healthcare industry is on track to make up as much as a third of the U.S. economy, this regulation and distribution are paramount.

The medical profession is one that, for its size and scope, is a rather closed community. Due to their affluence, its members at one time practiced what became known as "professional courtesy," whereby other doctors and their immediate families would be serviced by their colleagues without charge, or at most, an automatic acceptance of the doctors' insurance coverage. That is changing. Now that physicians are feeling the tightness of the privately run third-party system that has seriously reduced their returns, and with the costs of doing medical business remaining at peak levels thanks to high rents, office salaries, overhead, and above all, ever-soaring medical malpractice premiums, more and more practitioners are reluctant to extend that courtesy. And with many clinicians refusing Medicare fees for their senior patients, even the geriatric doctor community has found itself unwelcome among friends.

As the nation's physicians were so very much a part of the resistance to national healthcare programs, a good deal of that resistance was their recalcitrance to being labeled as less than elegant professionals. There was objection to the sobriquets "tradespeople," "service agents," and "workers" or "employees," despite their being very much exactly that.

Medicine Joins the Union

More, from the Red-baiting climate of the twenties and thirties with those demonization ploys of "socialized medicine" altering our practice and thinking, to the McCarthy scares of the 1950s, unions and organized labor became associated with Vladimir Lenin, Joe Stalin, and "Godless" communism. That was to be avoided at all costs.

"Better dead than Red!" was still in. "No union for me!" was the doctors' battle cry.

This has happened elsewhere and for the same reasons and with the same convoluted thinking. During the height of the Cold War and the Red Scare mania, with McCarthyism at full momentum, while the American Medical Association (AMA) was using its wiles to encourage antipathy to organizing in order to protect their member doctors and the U.S. public from the bugaboo of socialized medicine, the House UnAmerican Activities Committee (HUAC), Senator McCarthy's aegis, took full aim at another U.S. institution—Hollywood and the American movie industry.

Memories are still vivid of the Hollywood inquisitions that paraded one star after the other, ferreting out the activists in the Screen Actors Guild (SAG) for "fellow travelers" that accused certain members of putting "Communist leanings" into screen plays and even insisted many were Communist Party members (some were). The "Hollywood 10" became a group of the industry's leading and most skilled writers who leaned on the Constitutional rights of the Fifth Amendment, protecting them from self-incrimination.

They didn't have to be indicted or convicted of breaking any law, of which there were none and which they did not. The blackballs were put into place and they became outcasts forever. Others sadly did not have such courage or honesty and became friendly witnesses for the HUAC. They suffered the disdain and scorn of their Hollywood colleagues.

But certainly one of the excuses given by those who turned against their co-workers as "stool pigeons" was the same one U.S. physicians and their AMA fell back on—that they did not want to be associated with anything so "left" or "Red" as a union, or being "organized" into worse than a union—a "trade union." Doctors were taught to consider themselves "above that."

In lieu of "union," Hollywood used the label "guild." Doctors were not "workers" or "tradespeople," they were "actors and actresses" who were on the same side as their producers and movie moguls and most, the HUAC. McCarthy and the HUAC counted on the turncoats in tinsletown to be sufficiently "above" those labels. That ploy worked as well as it had in U.S. medicine. The movie industry has never been the same.

But now that the doctors are at odds with the newly corporate takeover of healthcare in America, they find themselves very much in the roles of employee, worker, or members of a trade. I was a house officer in the mid-sixties. "Union" was then a dirty word; "strike" was scarier. Any hint at organization and you were labeled at least a "fellow traveler," or even worse.

We were then considered students, or just "student doctors." And that is the way we felt. After all, we were still learning our trade, no pun intended. The salaries, using a word that was also supposed to be avoided, were not a living wage. The hospitals preferred the word "stipend." We used to kid about it and say we worked for "'X' dollars a week and all we could steal." No, we did not commit real felonies. But we did learn to be prudent and resourceful.

The dining service would regularly send the meal trays for every patient up to the floors. There were some that we had ordered "nothing by mouth" in anticipation of the next morning's surgery, or as a monitored post-op recovery whose status did not allow for the standard food. We learned to pounce on those meals, waiting eagerly for the stacks of trays, finding the ones that were for the patient we had chosen to feed us and sneaking off to our quarters. The microwave had not yet been invented, so we had to improvise to heat up our dinners if they got cold while we completed our duties. There were always the autoclaves used for the sterilization of medical instruments. Somehow it all worked out. When you are young and eager, things do.

It was later in the '60s that the rumors of the 1950s came true house staffs throughout the country were actually organizing. It just got there a little too late for me.

The Committee of Interns and Residents (CIR) is the only meaningful and certainly the largest medical staff trade union in the country. It now represents over 12,000 house officers in California, Florida, Massachusetts, New Jersey, New York, Washington, DC, and Puerto Rico. Founded in 1957, it has made quite an impact.

In 1997, CIR affiliated with the 1.6 million-member Service Employees International Union (SEIU) that includes about 870,000 healthcare workers throughout the nation. No doubt that the "in unity there is strength" motto enhanced the bargaining power of both unions.

The anlage for CIR was in the New York City public hospital system. CIR bargained for its first labor contract with a hospital in 1958. After it was well established as the bargaining chip for house staffs by the end of that decade, members joined up from private, or voluntary, sectors. The Committee of Interns and Residents became a reality.

CIR has always been conscious of the danger of public scrutiny, knowing that citizens would look sternly on any group that would take a job action when their responsibilities so directly related to people's lives and health. That concern has never been ignored.

When there have been threats and walk-out fears, those obligations were never shirked. Never has a hospital been denied not only the minimum but also adequate coverage so that patient health and welfare have never been compromised in any way, shape, or form. Never. The Hippocratic oath has always taken precedent to any other priorities or issues.

The SEIU has now expanded to all those considered healthcare workers, and not only doctors and nurses. The add-ons include hospital security workers, janitors, home care workers, school workers, bus drivers, and nursing home workers.

Out of all this, as the medical community yielded and became "organized," physicians have become interested in other aspects of their political lives. At the highest of levels, many physicians have become directly involved in the politics of their communities and have run and gained elective offices. It is no coincidence that the present majority leader in the U.S. Senate and the newly elected president of the Democratic National Committee (DNC) are physicians. The DNC head, Howard Dean, MD, has already been a serious presidential aspirant and is showing signs that he will be once again in 2008. House and Senate bodies have a smattering of other doctors. Several states already have many physicians in their legislatures. At the last count, thirty state legislatures have MDs in office this past term.

Doctors, once somewhat myopic in their outlooks *vis à vis* politics, have spread well out beyond the absolute medical/scientific sector. As the CIR/SEIU started taking its place in the work scene, house staffs became more comfortable with some form of the moniker "organized labor." In a real sense, this new attitude is a part of what is behind their uprisings against being taken over by the banking and insurance combines.

The old timers out there who did their residencies and postgraduate training before the CIR was around are taking a back seat as a new wave of clinicians move into the private workplace and admit to the positive experience of inclusion in an organized workforce. I hope this will pay dividends in the years to come as these now private-sector doctors mobilize themselves to take back their profession.

The Medical Model in Society

As the economics behind the multi-layered medical industry are exposed and examined by the U.S. public, so, too, are the other mores of our social order that factor into the familiar structure. We can see other seeds of belief play into the choices of those college students who go on to medical school and enter the traditional world of medicine in this country. The lingering conceptions and myths, beliefs that were never true but will always be, seem to govern our lives in subtle ways.

We physicians, like the society from which we come, are not necessarily misogynist, but androcentric. We are not racist but Eurocentric. We are not anti-Semitic but Christocentric. We are not homophobic but heterocentric. We are not nationalistic but geocentric.

Women, therefore, as expected, have had the same difficulties entering the field of medicine as they have had in all other sectors of society. Of course, things are changing and progressing as our whole social order moves ahead. But, perhaps slower than we think.

In 2003, the last year reported, the differences in wages between males and females got wider, not narrower, despite doing the same job in the same industry. The same is also true, by the way, between black and white wages—differences increased.

But in 2003, for the first time in U.S. history, women outnumbered men in the ranks of medical school applicants. For the 2003–04 year, women represented 51 percent of the applicants, an almost 8 percent increase from the year before. And this was not a one-time event. This has been the trend over the past decade, also reflective of the turnaround in medical school applicants in general. The 1990s saw a decline in overall applications.

Likewise in graduating residents. For example, in obstetrics and gynecology, there is a definite trend toward female graduates. In 2003, 70 percent of all residents finishing accredited programs in the U.S. were women. While it is true that obstetrics has been a more female-oriented specialty, along with pediatrics and the non-clinical fields, such as pathology and radiology, there are signs that this is happening in all areas.

Such exclusively male specialties as general surgery and urology are also seeing changes. This is yet another area in which the U.S. is playing catch up to the rest of the developed world in both general medical studies and specialties. Other nations are seeing a greater influx of women applicants. In some specialties as high as 90 percent.

The slow but visible swing toward more people of color entering the field of medicine also reflects an overall trend. Before the advents of the sweeping and long overdue 1960s civil rights legislation that was culminated in the Bakke and Michigan Supreme Court decisions that strengthened affirmative action in graduate education, medicine was surely a white career. Just as there were obvious and well-documented quotas that limited Jewish students in medical school classes, African- American and Hispanic college premeds were considerably closed off from the medical schools, except for the two or three that were below the Mason-Dixon Line and even only accepted blacks. Certainly not yet equal to their percentages in the U.S. population, nonwhites are making some progress in medical school and residency training programs.

Marcus was a ruddy sixty-eight-year-old handyman in his ghetto neighborhood, well known and well loved by his friends and neighbors. His sudden episode of searing chest pain and dizziness that brought a 911 ambulance to his basement apartment worried everyone who had come to his aid. He was rushed to the nearest hospital.

Stabilized by the chief nurse and admitting ER officer, he was told to rest and wait for the chief resident in cardiology to take over his case. Marcus was now pain free and leaned back on the hospital cot to wait his turn.

A husky, square-jawed fellow with a polished look finally appeared, wearing a starched white doctor coat, a stethoscope in one pocket, and his very black hand in the other. He was obviously in command, drawing to attention the junior house attendant and nurses. He was handed Marcus' chart, started his read, and asked a few pertinent questions of his colleagues.

Marcus looked up, took in the scene, and asked an orderly standing by his bedside who that black fellow was. "That's Doctor Johnson, chief heart doc. He will see you in a minute," was the reply.

Marcus peered more attentively and called over his nurse.

"That guy," pointing to Doctor Johnson. "He's gonna take care of me?"

"Oh, yes," replied the nurse. "In a moment."

"No way," Marcus quickly answered back. "I know that guy. He's Danny Johnson's boy. I recognize him from my neighborhood. Don't know where he's been these past few years. Ain't seen him around much. But I want a real doctor, not that guy. No way."

The nurse smiled and assured Marcus that Doctor Johnson was indeed a real doctor and legitimate, the chief of the service and one of the best. Marcus was in good hands, he was told with an assuring pat on the shoulder.

"No way," insisted Marcus with a harsh tone to his voice. "No kid of Danny Johnson ever gets to be a doctor. No way is he gonna take me on. No way. I want a real one."

The denouement was that in order to relieve Marcus of his cultural concerns, Doctor Johnson, informed of Marcus' reaction, gave out a broad smile of his own and knowingly nodded to his second in command to take the Marcus case. ♦

Identifying with and relating to your doctor, in whose hands you are placing your life, play a major role in your success as a patient. Recovery and rehab depend upon more than pulse taking, EKG interpretation, a maze of laboratory results, the writing of a prescription, opening your mouth and saying "Ah," and the hi-tech toys doctors play with, which, when properly applied, are adapted to manage all patients, and not as a further widening of that schism between the haves and the have nots.

Healing is facilitated and achieved by an understanding of your pathology, an expectation of a triumph in your treatment, and an acceptance when there are reasonable setbacks. It is a feeling of comfort that you are in the secure charge of a trusted and knowing healer.

Physicians are molded, sculpted, honed, polished, and then spit-shined. The results are fellow human beings who, because of an investment by both doctor and patient, warrant the trust that comes from unique, satisfying exchanges called patient-doctor communication.

That is medicine practiced with a license. It is the only acceptable medicine people need and deserve.

CHAPTER 4

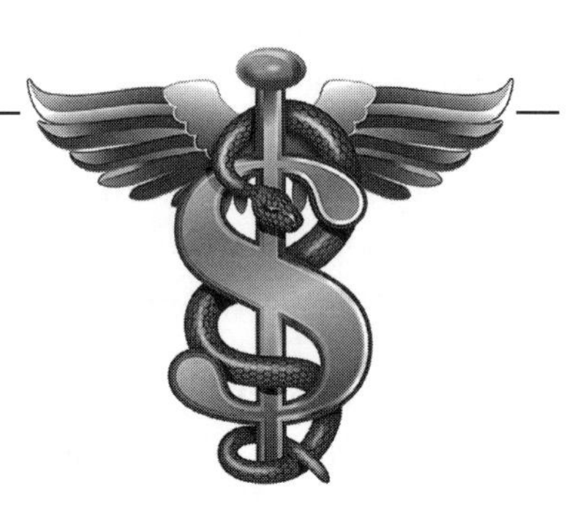

Socialized Medicine— A Commie Plot? The Ploy of Demonization

The Roosians are comin'! The Roosians are comin'!" That was followed by "The Vietcong are comin'! The Vietcong are comin'!" And now we have "The (fill in the blank) are comin'! The (fill in the blank) are comin'!" The "blank" is interchangeable—Arabs, Muslims, Iraqis, Iranians, terrorists, Palestinians, Syrians, Libyans, Cubans, or any combination thereof. Even Martians, if that suits its purpose. You know what they say. You've seen one, you've seen them all. The Russians were stereotyped with full fur-lined hats that looked a lot like helmets, with big earflaps that were only to be used when they were shipping off renegades to Siberia. "Siberia" and the gulags were made synonymous with "Hell," all as part of the demonization process.

The Vietnamese were dressed in khaki green and had protruding big teeth. Great care was taken to ensure this image was not confused with the depiction of the Japanese, who were now our trading partners and friends. During World War II, a very similar visage had been applied to the Japanese, then our enemy. The Middle Easterner's face was always shaded with a three-day beard growth. Of course, there was an Arafat-type *berneuse* and a partial cloth facemask. We once depicted Libyan President Muammar al-Quaddafi as one of our most villainous characters. He was accused of being a world-class criminal who blew up our airplane and killed countless numbers of our men, women, and children. Now we have extended him full diplomatic recognition with exchange of ambassadors. He is even shown as a public ally in Western dress and no five o'clock shadow. It all depends with whom we are doing business.

Our propaganda experts could have taken their lessons in that art of demonization from the AMA, which, back in the 1930s, started up what may be one of the most successful demonization campaigns of all time. The bugaboo? Socialized medicine. Any hint of a change in the way the USA practiced medicine, even the slightest suggestion that those who went without any care at all would be covered in some way, any way, by public assistance, invoked the cry, "Socialized medicine."

It was the word "socialized" that was intended to put fear into the hearts and minds of all good Americans who have been brainwashed to fear anything those "Roooosians" might import from behind the Kremlin walls. It was all very, very effective.

America's Image

American medicine stayed the way it was. The AMA was the self-anointed guardian of America's doctors and their way of life. The physician took on a stereotype of his/her own (mostly his in those days). The image came from that time-honored *Saturday Evening Post* Norman Rockwell cover that painted the scene of a Small Town, USA, doctor's office: the ancient-looking white male physician with a white beard, scraggly just enough to show that he was a hard-working soul who had probably been up all night sitting at the bedside of his needy patient, the family awestruck by his presence.

His white lab coat was waist-sized, and he peered at a nine-year-old lad over spectacles that were perched halfway down his nose. In his hand was a wooden tongue depressor, gently leaning down into his patient's gaping mouth, as he asked for the traditional "Ahhhh." Behind him stood his faithful nurse, of similar age. They were never cute and young in those days. She was coyly hiding the hypodermic syringe under her white smock, while the family doc was preparing the little boy for what we all knew had to come.

A cherry lollipop on the doctor's desk completed the picture, all designed to show that ol' Doc Whoever was like a second dad. Every stick of the needle with that life-saving miracle drug was followed by the candy on a stick. Mama was sitting in the corner, eyes cringing, vicariously about to share her son's pain of the needle. There was no limit to how often we could show that portrait. It became emblazoned in our consciousness.

We were also led to believe, and many did, that money did not necessarily enter into the transaction. The ol' doc would take whatever you offered; it was implied. Somehow, we just never figured into the equation that he had to pay rent, the phone bill, liability insurance, and that nurse's salary. Somehow, it was just figured that his kids would go off to college and there was always someone, a male, of course, who would follow in his footsteps. That *Saturday Evening Post* cover image would live into eternity.

But this is no longer the 1930s. The world plunged into a global war that brought us jet airplanes, radar, computers, and satellites. Not only did we learn to predict the weather, our communication technology jumped ahead by light years. The Civil War was no longer being fought on the battlefield, and U.S. apartheid was getting shaken at its base. We came to realize that the U.S. was indeed a cosmopolitan nation of immigrants and the different nationalities and races have to learn to live as one.

Along with the creation of a UN and the economic structure known as Bretton Woods, our legacy from the morass that was World War II and the Holocaust was the concept of human and civil rights. Civil rights was "in," and in 1954, the Supreme Court's decision to desegregate schools (Brown v Board of Education) became the law of the land. We also learned that the segregation of colored and impoverished America was about more than just separate public bathrooms and neighborhoods. There was a class structure at work that served a purpose, restricting a people who would work for less, toil longer hours, and even be grateful for the chance. But when Jim Crow started to take the front seat in the bus, it came out that our nation was divided in many other subtle ways.

Brown v Board started us off on school desegregation. That was in the public domain. That was visible, and somehow, education—required by law up to a certain age—was not "private." Only the very wealthy went to private academies and ivy-walled classrooms. Middle class America stayed put for the most part, and with Brown v Board slow to implement, schools more than de facto stayed segregated. That jury is still out.

But medicine and our healthcare were not for public tampering. The AMA spent more and more of the doctors' dues on a demonization program that was intended to maintain the status quo.

A Changing World

In November 1917, Vladimir Lenin fired the cannon from the deck of the cruiser *Aurora,* anchored in the Neva River in then and now St. Petersburg, on the Czar's Winter Palace, signaling the onset of the Soviet Revolution. We had our built-in demon. Socialism. Better, communism, a more poignant scare word.

We were told that Karl Marx's opening line of his 1848 *Communist Manifesto* that predicted "a specter was haunting Europe, that specter is communism," was becoming reality. We were all told we had better stay alert. And when that Marxist experiment got underway in Russia, we learned of the complexity of the entity that was "socialism." It turned out to be some form of a forerunner to true Marxism or communism. No matter about the chronology. Here, socialism was enough of a demon. Even that would mean the end to our "American way of life." That is all we needed to know.

As that change in sociology and economics took hold in Russia, becoming the Soviet Union, the Soviet philosophers and enforcers first attacked and changed two systems—education and healthcare. The Russian peasants and underclass had U5MRs that rivaled those of sub-Saharan Africa. And the Soviet founders knew right off the importance of having a healthy and literate people if the revolution were to survive.

As a part of the process, everything they had became "socialist," from stores, factories, theatre, art, music, literature, and the military, to schools and medicine. Doctors became employees of the state, just like everybody else. Okay. We could accept socializing road builders, factory workers, and electricians to get higher wages and a few weeks' vacation. But doctors? Never. That would really be meddling with our precious "American way of life." Something had to be done.

Something was. The demonization process was put into motion. The USA was the best, we were told. Our doctors and medical schools and hospitals were the finest in the world. Why? Because there was that motivation of wealth and the prestige that went with it that was associated with the physician in private practice. What did every boy and even girl eventually want to grow up to be? An Oscar-winning movie star, a trophy-awarded professional athlete, and...a doctor.

Never mind that already millions of American citizens were without any healthcare at all. In the South, with segregated hospitals, as well as washrooms and restaurants, public clinics and emergency rooms were put at the disposal of the disenfranchised—only if the public budgets allowed for them.

As more black doctors managed to find their ways into the nation's medical schools, still quite segregated, more African-Americans became exposed to the marvels of private medicine. To have your own doctor meant a mark of accomplishment and success. The trouble was there were just not enough to go around, and the system would never allow for it, anyway.

There was then that specter that was haunting America—the specter of integration, the beginning of the end of racism and Jim Crow. And, as schools started to open up (never mind the reality that was a segregation system that holds to this very day with the influx of private academies and classrooms), medicine was next. The harsh truth became more evident: U.S. healthcare was now our worst disgrace. And there were rumbles that something had to be done. Unrest among the people reached new heights.

But the AMA held on. It had taught the U.S. physician community that their very culture, prestige, and place in our economy were being threatened. Socialized medicine was named as the alternative, and nothing was worse than that. That is what they had in the Kremlin and in "Godless" communist Russia. The doctors took the bait, hook, line, and sinker. They just gladly paid the dues increase to the AMA and held on for dear life. It was an easy sell.

America went into a funk after the glitzy age of the "Roaring Twenties." The mood swings of our economy took a nosedive. October 1929 was looming. Factories were turning out goods and products that were beyond the pocketbooks of the working people of America. The materials backed up on the shelves and in the warehouses.

Europe had not yet recovered from World War I, and famine and homelessness became the rule of the day. Markets dried up. Wall Street just could not cover its losses, and the market dropped through the cellar. The bailout got underway. Never mind that the system had failed. Someone had to take the fall. Who else but the president? After all, it happened on his watch. Herbert Hoover took the hit.

The New Deal

The United States then entered a momentous era, one that saw the recovery from the Great Depression, the remarkable turn about of the U.S. political system to one of marked government involvement, World War II, the post-war recovery, and the Cold War with the eventual fall of the USSR. This was all due to the inauguration of the New Deal, the catch phrase of Franklin Delano Roosevelt (FDR) who became a four-term president and left in his wake a set of institutions and laws that have become the standard by which the USA is identified.

Thus came the union shop, minimum wage, workman's compensation, unemployment insurance, old age pensions, Social Security, graduated income tax, banking rules that included certain drastic regulations that are still intact. Government construction projects in all then forty-eight states. The Tennessee Valley Authority (TVA) that brought electricity to the South and job camps and government-sponsored work units, some of which were shown to be unconstitutional, set the pace before they were declared so and discarded.

They put America back to work. FDR took the partly coincidental retirements and deaths on the Supreme Court to "pack" it with those justices who were in consort with his plans for recovery. Arguably, the New Deal was perhaps the most dynamic changeover in government in our history. Only the Civil War and that decade in Vietnam are its rivals. We are waiting to see how our Iraqi adventure stacks up when future history books are written.

But, as wide-ranging as it was, healthcare for the most part, except by attrition, did not budge. The AMA managed to keep the American medical institution away from FDR's knife and pen. Health insurance for all was always kept on a back burner, despite the remarkable changes effectuated in just about all other areas of the social order. In fact, no one ever seemed to ask about it.

Many historians of the era have claimed that they are unable to find writings or positions officially taken by FDR himself on the issue. Perhaps it was just that the AMA and the medical institution were that well entrenched. Or perhaps, I'd like to think, he was just so occupied with salvaging the nation at large he was not able to apply himself to everything.

Arthur J. Altmeyer, often called "The Father of Social Security," was a member of Roosevelt's inner circle. As a member of FDR's Committee on Economic Security (CES), the think tank that conjured up many of those brilliant populist programs that have become U.S. icons, he was at the forefront of many of the New Deal blueprints.

Altmeyer claimed that FDR almost felt compelled to avoid the issue of healthcare, though he knew how it was needed. The president's personal contact was through his son, Jimmy, whose father-in-law was the eminent Harvard neurosurgeon and researcher Harvey Cushing. Cushing and FDR had many a personal private fireside chat over the issue of healthcare, and apparently the power and position of the AMA were often raised.

Eleanor Roosevelt, FDR's influential activist wife, had often expressed concerns that the quality of healthcare that was being delivered under the private system would diminish if left to a government health insurance plan. Eleanor's inner circle included those who were of the same mind, and they always urged a hands-off attitude.

Altmeyer also recounted that the CES brought up the matter at one meeting and the president indicated he wanted to table it, claiming that a clash with the AMA and a well-contented community of American physicians would be unwise and unrewarding. Altmeyer insisted that Roosevelt never made this a formal request, but that the drift from the president was clear. As the CES was putting the finishing touches on the Social Security bill, which did have a space for a healthcare codicil, it was excluded as a matter of course. The Altmeyer Amendment was semiofficially tabled.

One of the most influential, if not the most influential, member was the Secretary of Labor, the Cabinet's first female ever, Frances Perkins. Secretary Perkins had rightly been given credit for much of the New Deal populist thinking that stemmed out of her own very progressive background and philosophy. When she implored the Committee, Altmeyer, and her boss to indeed add a healthcare rider to the Social Security presentation to Congress, FDR replied that Social Security itself would be a tough fight up on the Hill, and that it should not be imperiled by any contaminating healthcare additives. "We got to fight the fights we can win," was attributed to FDR. Perkins always backed off. Her respect for Roosevelt was that great.

In his book on the era, *The Formative Years*, Altmeyer writes that after the bill went through an extensive debate on the floor of Congress with enough optimism for passage, the Perkins rider could have been added as an afterthought, in hopes to slide it by. But the president was content enough to get Social Security through on its own merit, and its significance was too great. He did not wish to endanger the bill with more debate.

Part of the problem was a time constraint. Congress was about to adjourn for the summer recess in July of 1934, and the intricacies of adding that health bill portion would have delayed it for perhaps another year. Altmeyer insisted as well that the CES intended to keep the matter of that truant healthcare issue alive to be tackled the following year. A debate raged in committee over a secondary and perhaps stop gap bill to at least pass catastrophe coverage. But that was soon dismissed when even the proponents of total coverage claimed that this would be settling for something that was still far too insufficient for the people's needs. Altmeyer wrote that the CES was hoping for a change of heart by their medical advisory subcommittee that was working on the AMA and the medical community spokespersons. No such luck.

The AMA remained adamant and steadfast. They wanted hands off by big government. This was mostly the work and influence of the AMA president and journal editor (1924–49), the legendary Missourian Doctor Morris Fishbein, a name that became synonymous with the American Medical Association and its struggle to keep U.S. medicine private. The commercial insurance conglomerates remained strangely in the background, sensing all along that they had sufficiently demonized any form of governmental interference in healthcare as "socialized," and that was that. The Kremlin's shadow was still lurking.

Fishbein and the AMA upstaged organized labor, now so much better entrenched by many of the New Deal statutes that protected the union shop. Unions did not have the powered energy to combat organized medicine with any sort of campaign for healthcare for working America. Many historians of the period express surprise that the burgeoning CIO and AFL, fast becoming labor's voice, did not indicate any interest in this issue. Perhaps they realized they could not stack up against the Fishbein/AMA task force.

Perkins and her followers, including Altmeyer on this issue, did not just throw in the towel completely. In 1937, the CES made a second stab for healthcare. As the midterm election of 1938 was on the horizon, his secretary of labor grabbed President Roosevelt's attention and he reconvened the committee. He agreed that it might just be the right year to introduce such a thing as healthcare to the voting public. Just might.

But in the final push, the pleas fell on deaf ears, and FDR remained convinced that it was better politics to await the 1940 presidential campaign. Then history stepped in. The Hitler juggernaut was exploding in Europe and the entire world felt threatened. Suddenly, the thought-to-be lame duck president became an unprecedented third-term candidate.

Rumbles from Abroad

The talk of war was everywhere. Neville Chamberlain, the British Prime Minister, gave his infamous "peace in our time" speech and Adolf Hitler began gobbling up the European continent. The president of the United States kept making the partly logical excuse that he had other things on his mind than that elusive healthcare that never seemed to get past the drawing board.

As the CES and FDR were jockeying for position, the healthcare additive would not go away. Some form of disability insurance for on the jobbers did get enough White House notice to go through some hot and heavy debate. In private, at least, disability insurance was never thought to be a Social Security deal breaker. It seemed, for a moment, to have a jump-start. After all, FDR was told, any guy who had enough clout to get a third term over a formidable and strong candidate was ready for just about anything. But trouble reared up before long. The status quo reigned.

Altmeyer and his Oval Office boss were content to let the Social Security board handle the fight. By the time 1939 came around, Europe was even more of a powder keg waiting to explode. Healthcare was put off another year, administrative problems given as the excuse. By this time, commercial insurance companies, heretofore silent, lined up with the AMA and offered some cash benefits to those disabled on the job. That helped to quiet down the New Dealers.

Without the roaring energy and verve of the CES and the White House voice, even that kept getting postponed. The president took sides, completed a major sale of destroyers to Great Britain, and Lend

Lease was in full force. The predictable Wehrmacht invasion of Poland came in the fall of 1939, and 1940 saw the almost unimaginable crushing of the Maginot Line, the fall of France, and the Battle of Britain. Not only London was visited by the Luftwaffe every night. Europe was literally up in flames. That took all the attention FDR could muster.

Then came December 7, 1941, and the USA was at war.

Congressional Denials

Enter Wagner-Murray-Dingell. The original 1943 W-M-D bill introduced by Robert Wagner, Democrat senator from New York, was meant to attach a national health insurance rider to Social Security, which was already established and accepted since 1935 as one of the great progressive achievements in U.S. history.

Social security and other programs were making serious inroads into American life. Everybody wanted to jump on the bandwagon. Congress introduced statutes for unemployment compensation and general federal relief for emergencies and catastrophes. W-M-D, however vague and somewhat shallow, provided a basis for a national healthcare and hospitalization fund to which employees and employers would contribute.

The self-employed would make their contributions in the same way. There were also some disability provisions, coverage for laboratory tests, and X-rays (although dental, nursing, and medications were not included). The national fund was then to be used to pay physicians and hospitals for any services rendered through a combination of fee-for-service or capitation.

There was mass support for the bill from organized labor and many community organizations, especially from middle America. The consensus was clear. It was considered such a vast improvement over the wonted scant coverage that it was a puzzlement by many as to how and why anyone would not support it.

There were those forces that felt the federal government would have to play the major role if this were to be a success. There was a fear that by relying on the states to carry out the plan, too many bargaining chips would be introduced and fat cats and local pols would get into the act and destroy the original purpose—to provide the nation with a national healthcare plan it so desperately sought.

There was enough of a track record to show that this could happen. Federal unemployment insurance and other forms of public assistance had been in operation for two years or more. The Great Depression had created the need for such measures. But there were many signs that state-level mechanisms and administrations just could not get the job done. The feds kept moving into the act of all of the New Deal programs and taking hold of the reigns of control. Then there was that concern at the top, in Roosevelt's Administration, that the AMA and private practitioners together were strong enough to fight the advent of any state-level public services and easily undermine any program if not closely watched by Washington. FDR and his inner loop decided that if W-M-D or any program of that nature were to be enacted, it would have to be under strict federal controls.

And there was that very vociferous mass opposition spawned by the Fishbein nucleus apart from the general hostility at the AMA. That was the exact time that the demonization PR moved into high gear. "Socialized medicine" was first introduced as a term, and it did a number on the U.S. medical community and their patients. Some of the billboards and full-page ads featured a doctor or hospital scene being choreographed by a Russian bear with gritting teeth.

The demonization campaign painted a picture that doctors would be working for the federal government on a nine-to-five workday. If you got sick after hours—tough on you. You would just have to wait until the doctor checked in the next working day. Weekends and holidays? Forget about it! That lovable old man pictured on the *Saturday Evening Post* cover was rocking away on his front porch. You would just have to "take two aspirin and call me in the morning."

The PR was very effective. The people would be turning over their well-being to the U.S. Surgeon-General and the U.S. Public Health Service. But, what those entities were never was clearly understood. Bright red brochures and pamphlets filled every doctor's waiting room, crying out against the abomination of turning over their docs and their care to big government, like the "Rooosians" did under the guide of Vladimir Lenin or Joe Stalin. "Socialized medicine" was inserted at every opportunity. Ad nauseum. But it caught on.

The funny part about it was that the W-M-D bill had such good intentions—the start of a system to give all Americans some form of healthcare. Even those who were obviously from the violent opposition publicly admitted that the U.S. population was deserving of a national healthcare package and that W-M-D was a good way to break the ice. But we all know what the road to hell is paved with. The bill did not recommend any provisions for assigning patients to doctors, and no regulations for doctors' hours or payments, compensations for facilities or supplies, or a means of doctor coverage and assistants.

There were no allowances for hospital construction that would surely be needed if Americans were to go from being potential to real patients. It actually encouraged that Norman Rockwell image, as though all those family docs would be able to carry the load.

In fact, even some of its staunchest supporters, save Wagner and Murray and Dingell, expressed sharp and public doubts as to its worth in the long run. They were concerned that only employed persons would be covered, with no protection for those between jobs or the unemployable. And it finally got mentioned that maybe W-M-D was far too centralized, without enough state and local participation. But it was a start. At the time, it was certainly worth fighting for.

The legal community eventually put their two cents in, even though this was as yet an era before medical malpractice moved into high gear. The American Bar Association (ABA) became part of the opposition. It made the point that W-M-D did not provide for a court review of any future administrative decision (as though that *were* meaningful at the time).

The whole thing became so convoluted that even Altmeyer, FDR's champion on this issue, waffled. With the president wavering, as well, and with the turmoil in Europe building up to the boiling point, there was little energy left to deal with this pressing issue at home, especially when the opposing forces were so well organized. Altmeyer admitted in his memoirs that he never actually endorsed the W-M-D bill in all its details. That became evident when the committee never held a roll-call vote and its report to Congress never specifically endorsed the bill about to come before it.

Blame was switched from hand to toe. The Bureau of the Budget was dumped on for not getting its analysis back in time, so full support and that endorsement was never given because the bill had to have those costs and statistics to give the whole story. The campaign for W-M-D was in shambles.

One contrasting moment and conundrum in political history rose up in the role of Sam Rosenman, a most trusted FDR advisor, confidante, and close personal friend.

One vignette has Judge Rosenman rise bright and early every Saturday morning from his upper west side New York apartment, and have his driver stop off at Barney Greengrass, the city's legendary dairy deli, for a supply of bagels, cream cheese, and smoked salmon. Then Rosenman hopped the Penn Station to DC's Union Station express in time to brunch with FDR in the Oval Office, along with the president's core brain trust—Cabinet heavies like Jim Farley from Post Office, Henry Wallace from Commerce, Harold Ickes from Interior, and, of course, Perkins from Labor, who made the real hard core decisions that ran the nation.

Judge Rosenman was strongly in favor of W-M-D, and along with Secretary Perkins, they never let up on their boss. With FDR's untimely death in April 1945, then-President Harry S. Truman had Rosenman stay on as advisor and speechwriter—eventually much to Truman's regret. Perkins and Wallace resigned almost immediately.

They eventually split widely on many political aspects, from the Cold War to healthcare. Perhaps Truman sincerely wanted to carry on with many parts of the New Deal, but he instead succumbed to the Cold War junkies, and the post-war period became just too complex.

The American Medical Association eventually won the final battle and the war. They had the funding to fight to the end. That demonization ploy was a very effective tool to win over the doctors, and there was seemingly no limit as to how much they would kick in as individuals and a group to lobby Washington against any form of "socialized medicine." Wagner, Murray, and Dingell became scare words and a virtual battle cry, along with "socialized medicine." Labor's organized support of the bill just could not outweigh what the medical community mustered up.

The fight for W-M-D didn't officially end. No one threw in a proverbial towel. The Social Security people continued to urge its passage. Little pieces of the plan were recommended separately, to no avail. Hospital benefits, for example, had been urged during the war in 1942. Even some hospital construction that was so acutely needed was promoted. To no avail. Other compromises were tried. Even Truman gave some subtle support.

It became evident that a national healthcare bill was not ever going to fly. Or so it seemed. In his memoirs, Altmeyer expressed many regrets and took the blame for its eventual failure.

Post-War USA

Move forward to late 1945. V-E and V-J days celebrations were waning, at least to a point that we could start to think and ponder our peacetime needs. The second version of the W-M-D bill was introduced into Congress in an attempt by its supporters to meet the criticisms of the earlier legislation. President Truman sent a message later that year urging the federal government to make some noise about healthcare. He did want to sound like a New Dealer; he just didn't know how to play the part very well without Franklin Delano Roosevelt and the brain trust at the helm.

Truman sounded specific, but in reality he was as vague as the rest. The AMA's threat and voice still rang loud and clear. Truman suggested some monetary benefits to cover time lost on the job during infirmities, expanding Social Security indices to include some health and even dental care, allowing funding for new hospital and clinic construction. He supported medical research and education, and even made specific plans to update and improve maternal-child healthcare programs.

Nothing seemed to help.

It appears that the president tried to cover all his bases and critics. Court reviews were written into the new law to assuage the ABA. There were nursing homes added, and other dental services were written into the bill. Although many state and local responsibilities were tagged on at the end, it was clear that the federal machinery would stay in control. The aegis of the Oval Office made an impression. And the supporters of the bill were willing to compromise in order to get something up to the Hill and on the floor that could come to a vote and have a real chance of passing.

That never happened. Senators Wagner and Murray and Representative Dingell seemed to be willing to rewrite their original legislation of 1943 into Truman's mold. They knew all along they were up against a good fight and seemed willing and anxious to do what had to be done to save the legislation as long as principle was not violated.

But even that didn't get it done. It just seemed too loosely connected. Grass roots supporters, from the masses of people and doctors and healthcare professionals, never forced the issue, claiming it was never clear who was in charge and how the finances would be managed. Most disheartening, they were alarmed that there were no actual obligatory provisions for doctors to join up.

The Hill-Burton Hospital Construction bill was introduced along with the renewed and revised W-M-D in 1945, but never got off the ground. This was simply intended to provide the states with building monies for hospital construction, and did indeed say that more would be allocated by the feds for poorer neighborhoods. This led to infighting between the states as to which would get the big bucks from DC. There would be federal guidelines for each state to follow, no matter if the hospital were to be a proprietary or a public institution.

Local communities would not be granted federal construction funds if they could not prove they would be able to support the hospital after opening. That was a tall order. This, in a way, was meant to assure that no white elephants would be constructed through some hanky-panky nepotism rulings and by "well-connected" people. This was one of the major reasons why the majority of Washington urged for as strict a federal control as possible. It was always felt that the more local the involvement and control, the more the chance for underhanded dealing and extortion. There was likely a good deal of truth to those concerns. Need, thus, had to be proved.

There was as well a fear that hospitals would be built in catchment areas where the residents would not be able to afford their maintenance while still others would blossom in areas of affluence but not have enough population or need to support their facilities. A catch-22 over and over.

The Wagner-Murray-Dingell bills never even came to a vote on the floor of Congress. They became history and were put to rest in the Congressional Record for posterity.

The AMA and privatization won.

Demonization was the weapon.

The American people lost.

The history books of the twentieth century easily tell the rest of the story. Healthcare took a back seat to what was happening in a post- war world. Europe had been decimated. The Holocaust was exposed for the entire world to see its horror. It became more evident daily just how treacherous were the Nazi regime and its gangster allies. The brutality of its genocide was too stark to be dinner table conversation.

America started to count its blessings and be grateful it was thousands of miles away from the death camps. Who had time to think about healthcare? We were just glad to be alive and intact and getting most of our soldiers home in one piece. Not all, just most. We were grateful and rightly so.

President Truman and his Joint Chief of Staff Commander, General George C. Marshall, donning civvies, concocted the European Recovery Act, better known as the Marshall Plan (MP). It got immediate funding and support.

Aimed mostly at Greece and Turkey, countries that had strong Communist Parties and were leaning toward the Soviet sphere of influence, the MP became ubiquitous and included just about any European nation that needed funds, food, and building supplies, in its determination to fend off any election that would take on a left shift. As Secretary of State Henry Kissinger would say a generation later, we were not about to sit idly by as a country was foolish enough to vote in a socialist government. That "Roooosians are comin'!" cry did not fade away. The East and the West divided up Europe and established their bases of power. PR and propaganda.

Roosevelt's New Dealer pal, Secretary of the Navy Frank Knox, died suddenly in 1944, and an apparently already weary FDR moved Under Secretary James Forrestal up a notch. In 1947, Truman promoted him to Secretary of Defense. Forrestal was a Joe McCarthy ally and equally as rabid in his determination to find a Commie in every corner and under every desk and in every drawer at the Pentagon.

Rumors of tax evasion brought an investigation into the Secretary's tax portfolio, which was found to include German/Nazi investments. Dismissed when his anti-Red mania reached a pinnacle of hysteria and distorted his job performance, Forrestal, paranoid and depressed, was admitted to the psychiatric service at the naval hospital in Bethesda. On May 22, 1949, Secretary of Defense Forrestal woke from his sleep in the middle of the night, donned his silk robe and slippers, and ran down the hallway screaming, "The Roosians are comin', the Roosians are comin'!" He leapt from a fifth floor window to his death. His suicide told us how far demonization could go. He believed his own hype. ♦

The Cold War and McCarthyism

British Prime Minister Winston Churchill started barn storming the United States and declared the Cold War. The nation's attention turned to stopping socialism in more ways than just in medical care. A lot of other people picked up the socialized label that worked so well for the AMA and the defenders of the private medical community.

Joe McCarthy became a household name; "McCarthyism" was emblazoned into our lexicon. Indeed, it is still there. We started protecting America from the socialization of Hollywood, the theatre, art, union shops, and government service in any areas that were deemed tainted. Everybody started taking loyalty oaths. We hadn't socialized medicine; we were not about to socialize anything else, either.

The United States was recovering from a wartime mode. We had passed out of the "Roaring and Glitzy" Twenties, using the New Deal and the miracles of FDR to get us past the Great Depression. That all had to be tabled in order to meet the responsibilities of the war. After all, with Europe in such an abyss, we were the suppliers of materials for use on the battlefields.

After Pearl Harbor, we had to take on a two-front war. No problem. We did indeed mobilize our factories and farms to provide the Allied forces with food, clothes, houses, and arms. And then we found enough left over to finance the Marshall Plan, one of the most remarkable undertakings in world history.

After the combined unconditional surrenders, many people assumed that the country would pick up where it had left off. And healthcare could assume some sort of priority. But that didn't happen.

The Cold War that President Truman endorsed with glee kept the nation in a wartime modus operandi. The U.S. stayed at a wartime pitch, and with the same conceived enemy—the Soviet Union and its experiment with socialism. There was just no shooting or body bags.

The Morris Fishbein era at the AMA started to fade away, although it was felt that his victory would be long lasting. Private USA medicine had been defended and it survived. As Europe recovered and their economies strengthened, just about all of what became the G-7 nations adopted one form or another of national health services. Great Britain and its former colony, Canada, paved the way, but the others followed suit. They bore different signatures, but the people all got covered. America remained mired into its Fishbein/AMA model. The U.S. health scene was going nowhere.

The Era Called Vietnam

Then history, as always, took over again. From out of the rubble came Korea, and, far worse, Vietnam. America entered what is arguably the worst decade in its history, perhaps rivaled only by its Civil War a century before. (Some political historians are starting to add the infamous Iraqi invasion of 2001 to that list.) Not only did Vietnam happen, but also Dallas happened, and no adult alive today has ever lived through a greater shock.

But just as President John F. Kennedy was lost, Martin Luther King, Jr., and his civil rights movement, sure to impact education and, down the road, the whole concept of healthcare, rose to the occasion. The opening of medical schools to black candidates changed the name of the game. New schools were founded. More doctors were being trained, and thus the patient to doctor ratio was improving. It was a foreshadowing of things to come.

The campaign of JFK had been a turning point in U.S. political history. U.S. politics was greeted by an Irish Catholic with a real electoral machinery, something the first of his faith, Al Smith, back in the '20s, lacked.

"Taking orders from the Pope" and other ugly negative campaign talk became the hustings rhetoric of the day. John F. Kennedy was also considered one of those "northeast liberals" who would run the country from a Boston country club. But the Kennedy clan was blossoming to create our first royal family, and Camelot became a reality.

The Kennedy platform included healthcare proposals, mostly of a routine nature. It seemed like politics as usual. But after the loss of hope in the years following the Truman dalliance with healthcare and the legacies of Wagner-Murray-Dingell, it was assumed that the "northeast liberal from Cambridge" would finally get serious about it. In fact, that was used as a campaign diatribe against the Kennedy platform; opponents rekindled the specter of "socialized medicine."

But history plays tricks in so many ways. The search for a 1960 vice-presidential slate partner demanded that there be a counter balance to the "Irish Catholic from Boston." That meant a Midwesterner, with good old U.S. American traditions. Ergo came the senator from Texas, Lyndon B. Johnson.

The alleged hayseed rancher with a Texas drawl moved into the Oval Office after JFK took his fateful trip down Dealy Plaza past the book depository in Dallas on November 22, 1963, and all of America thought we were in for the long ride of mediocrity, seen with Texans in the tradition of longhorn rancher Sam Rayburn running the show an era earlier. However, we were all in for a pleasant surprise.

On the international front, sadly, LBJ picked up the gauntlet from JFK and expanded that horror that was Indochina in a decade of tragedy that cost the lives of perhaps millions of Vietnamese, spread Agent Orange and other chemicals, and, of course, caused 58,000 U.S. soldier casualties that is a shame from which we have still not recovered.

The Vietnam War legacy includes homelessness, joblessness, hard-core drug abuse, AIDS, and the street crime that supports them all. Some 5 million troops rotated through Vietnam, 500,000 there at its peak, and from which we mustered out some 600,000 hard-core drug addicts, users, and sellers that came back to our inner cities. Without jobs, schools, or that ever-elusive healthcare, they were thrust into the mainstream society that shunned them, likely out of the guilt for having sent them there in the first place.

That wrangler from Texas also picked up some of the obviously popular programs that Kennedy was tragically denied enough time in office to carry out. However, LBJ apparently had no intention to maintain the team of advisors and cabinet officers that his slain predecessor had put together. Brother Bobby Kennedy as Attorney General and other lights from John Kennedy's Boston political family soon found themselves at odds with the new president, and it became more and more evident that candidate Johnson had indeed been a compromise with the Democratic soothsayers who never figured on November 22 and Dealy Plaza. The makeover of the Administration was swift and complete. Lyndon B. Johnson was determined to restore it in his image.

But there was a silver lining in that dark cloud: the country was finally given the first serious attempt at universal healthcare for at least two groups that were the most exposed and in need—the poor and the elderly. And this not from the Harvard liberal but from a Texas conservative.

Who could figure?

The Johnson Administration hatched Medicare and Medicaid, and despite their many shortcomings, they proved to be a start upon which the forces that were continually working for universal healthcare for all had to build. Wagner and Murray and Dingell would have been smiling. Their legacy had finally bore fruit. The ploy of demonization and those scare words, "socialized medicine" were still very much in use. And with the Cold War approaching its historical peak, the fear of the Kremlin was invoked by the forces of the right at every opportunity. Morris Fishbein was long gone, but his shadow still chilled the American medical community.

Just as FDR had felt the sting an era or two before and stayed away from a healthcare package for all rather than buck the AMA-rigged forces, American doctors were steeped in the security that government would never interfere with medicine as an industry. Yes, the very poor and even our senior citizens could have their programs; just leave the private doctor wearing that Norman Rockwell façade to his own wares. And yes, medicine was still a male career.

What has happened since? It has been wisely written by politicos, philosophers, journalists, and fiction and nonfiction writers that the turmoil of the '60s is unmatched in any other time frame in U.S. history.

The U-2 reconnaissance plane incident with Gary Powers led to the cancellation of the Paris peace conference in 1961 that might have put a serious dent in the Cold War. The Cuba crisis and the Bay of Pigs in a failed attempt to overthrow a Communist encampment in the western hemisphere. The eventual standoff between President Richard Nixon and Soviet Premier Nikita Khrushchev and the dismantling of the Soviet missiles in Cuba. The full escalation of the presidential war in Vietnam after the passing of the Gulf of Tonkin resolution that later on proved to be a deliberate untruthful exaggeration by the Johnson Administration.

The assassinations of Medgar Evers, John and Robert Kennedy, and Martin Luther King, Jr. Edward Brooke's election as the first black senator in eighty-five years and Thurgood Marshall's appointment as the first black Supreme Court justice in our history. The marches on Washington. The rioting and disruption of the 1968 Democratic convention in Chicago that led to a series of trials and court decisions and rewrote the laws on such future actions. The first moonwalk.

This indeed was quite a decade.

And there were Medicaid and Medicare. Of all the firsts in the period, these are undoubtedly the ones that should head the list of people-positive achievements.

It was felt, with certain credibility, that Medicaid and Medicare were enough for one year, one decade, some felt, one lifetime. For the first time in the history of the U.S., we actually had a federally funded and administered healthcare program for those otherwise denied. Just like the rest of the developed world.

But the deficits remained. Millions of citizens were left without care, again pushed onto the back burner. After all, this was a country of free enterprise, capitalism, and private industry.

Washington showed that such vital services as electricity, water supply, and electronic communications would be crucially needed during times of emergency, and that they belonged under a special kind of governmental control over and above the various regulatory monopoly laws passed in the late nineteenth century. The public utilities were thus created.

Why this special designation? Because certain services, like communication, electric power, and potable water were so vital for the welfare of a nation that strict controls were necessary to ensure their continual flow during times of national emergency, perhaps from enemy attack, certainly from natural disasters.

One of the major triumphal moments of the FDR New Deal had been the conception and construction of the TVA, a power plant delivery system that provided the U.S. Southeast with electric power not seen there before. The TVA came into fruition because no private power company or conglomerate would undertake the project, always insisting that it would be so costly, a sufficient profit could never be turned. Roosevelt retorted that profit had nothing to do with it—the need to serve the people did. The TVA success story is one of the most dramatic ones in our history.

Yet, healthcare, along with education, never seemed to fall into that category of vital national need. The AMA/socialized medicine/Fishbein/doctor acquiescence always won out. The school systems were left up to the states. Colleges and universities for the most part remained in private hands. And healthcare, save that little-albeit meaningful-dent of Medicaid and Medicare, was left to the private purveyors. Millions upon millions still went without.

What happened in our history and particularly in the era of the New Deal that provided the nation with the means of recovery from the Great Depression has become the symbol by which the United States is marked and is envied by the rest of the world.

Just as all republics in the Western world, and even parts of the Third World, have borrowed statutes and philosophies from our Constitution. Many of these same countries have taken pages from our populist deeds like minimum wage, social security, old age pensions, unemployment benefits, etc.

But healthcare? The opposite. It is we who must now stand in awe of the others that took that further step and have guaranteed their peoples basic education at a university level and—healthcare.

In our increasingly small world, the price we are paying for the demonization of government-run, nonprofit healthcare is starkly evident. Jet travel, exchanges between peoples from vastly different cultures, plus the need to stay in daily contact in order to avoid the holocaust in this nuclear world, have all made our health problems so complex and potential, a provision of healthcare is a matter of life and death. AIDS, as just one example, although it is still unclear how this epidemic got started, likely came from another continent and was here in a proverbial nanosecond. Who knows what else is lurking? Anthrax? Herpes? SARS? Avian flu?

The history of the twentieth century has surely taught us that national healthcare is not debatable and yet was always missing from the debate as the country moved forward after the Great Depression.

We hope the worm is turning. We can no longer afford to be without universal healthcare. A people who are ailing are so costly to the system that good health becomes a savings. Ill health becomes a drain on society. Health becomes a boon. The evidence is overwhelming and incontestable.

Our greatest wealth is our health.

CHAPTER 5

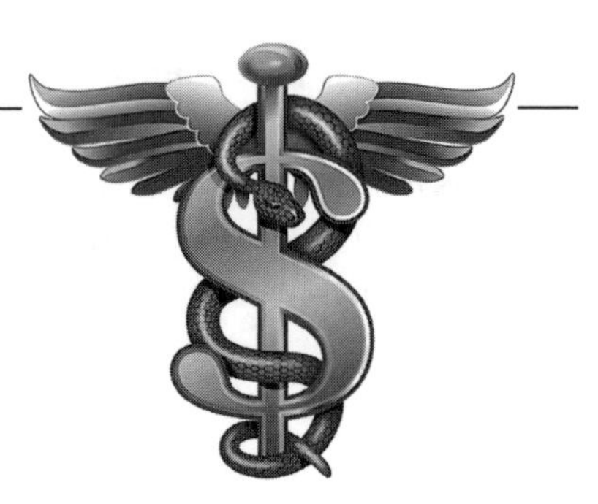

Medicare and Medicaid—The Only Shows in Town

Just to give you an idea of how bad off we are in this country, those of us working to promote a universal healthcare plan for everyone are finding ourselves fighting also to save Medicare and Medicaid, two flawed yet essential government-run care programs. Why? Because they are what we have to work with, and they are as good as we've ever known. And they are threatened. Without losing sight of the many needed changes, we must save them nonetheless. Thus, the healthcare movement has often been cornered into invoking the battle cry, "Medicare for all!" Because they are put in jeopardy year after year, we must start by protecting these programs, though we need so much more. Politics makes for strange bedfellows.

We must not fall into the trap of settling.

Medicare

Medicare is the current federal government service that helps provide healthcare for senior citizens and disabled Americans. Yes, it is available to all U.S. citizens over age sixty-five, but no, it does not provide total healthcare coverage. Not even close. It is broken down into two parts—Part A for hospital costs and Part B for doctor/medical costs. Part B requires a fee by the member. Free it ain't.

Medicare began back in the days of the New Deal and the Altmeyer/Perkins attempts to push through some form of healthcare for everyone within the FDR Social Security legislation in 1935. And, although the Franklin Delano Roosevelt think tank did their darnedest to slip it by a resistant Congress, it was abandoned for fear of losing the whole SS program. The rest of the 1930s saw all forms of healthcare tossed about as a political football from one Congressional committee to another, but none ever reached either body of Congress for full debate. It seems that every year there were national health conferences held in Washington that always closed with the issuing of recommendations to the White House urging the president move forward on a national health service. That was as far as they ever got. The Morris Fishbein AMA matched them committee for committee and always won.

It was in the president's State of the Union Address (SOTU) in 1943 that he first gave out his famous plea for social insurance "from the cradle to the grave" and added that we have the "right to adequate medical care and…the opportunity to enjoy good health." These statements were repeated in the SOTU's of 1944 and 1945, but sadly, most domestic programs were put on the back burner as the nation's attention was directed to a winding down of the war. FDR never made any specific suggestions to Congress. Even he was not about to take on the AMA. And, as we now look back, the president's personal health was so compromised by that time and going downhill faster and faster under the pressure to conclude the war, that he was dead three months later.

In the fall of 1946, the new President Harry S. Truman suggested a revival of the Wagner-Murray-Dingell bill and another attempt called the Taft-Smith-Ball bill that authorized grants to states for some forms of medical care, at least for the poor. But neither ever got to the floor for a vote. Senators Wagner, Murray, and Taft reintroduced their bills in 1947, but no action was taken. The debate on the floor included a sprinkling of the words "socialized medicine," meaning that the demonization ploy was still alive and effective.

The Congressional Record notes that in 1951, the annual Social Security Administration (SSA) report recommended that Congress take up some form of healthcare program for the country. But that is as far as it got—a recommendation without any introduction.

It took a back seat in public, at least, for the next several years. In 1960, under the name of Kerr-Mills, the SSA managed to get enacted a law that allowed for some funding to the states for healthcare. But the wording was imprecise and it was largely ignored and later shown to be devoid of any adequate teeth for implementation. Funding sources were, as usual, ambiguous, and the machinery was never put into place. More conferences convened in Washington, but they never got any further than the cosmetics.

It was President-elect John Kennedy, on the day after his election in November 1960, who appointed one Wilbur J. Cohen and formed a "Task Force on Health and Social Security for the American People." The committee specifically advocated some form of healthcare coverage for the aged. In 1961, with the advent of Camelot and the all-too-brief Kennedy era, the president sent messages to Congress and even took to network TV from Madison Square Garden in New York to make his plea for attention to the "Health of the Nation." This included the word "Medicare" for the first time. That was as far as it got. End of story. Private activists and most all of the minor political parties included healthcare in their platforms and chided the majors for the omission, but things went no further.

The gauntlet that was carried by the more liberal administrations of Roosevelt, Truman, and Kennedy was picked up by the cowpoke from Texas, Lyndon Baines Johnson. The senator was a well entrenched pol, steeped in the tradition of Texan Sam Rayburn, the powerhouse Aggie who rose to become the Speaker of the House for twenty-one years (1940–61) until his death, and gave the Lone Star State a real presence up on Capitol Hill that has, apparently, never waned to this very day. When the so-called Harvard-intellect from Boston was labeled too extreme an Eastern liberal, the story goes that he accepted a cracker from Texas as a running mate to give the Democratic Party a balanced ticket, never figuring on that fateful ride down Dealy Plaza in Dallas that allegedly changed the thrust of the Oval Office 180 degrees.

THE LEGACY OF LBJ

LBJ cleaned house in a hurry. Within a matter of months, Camelot's inner loop took on a new look. He used the terms coined by JFK, however, and again asked Congress to address the "Health of the Nation" in one speech after the other. On February 10, 1964, he officially named the advocated program "Medicare" and urged Congressional response. The Ways and Means Committee voted again to postpone action. Though their recommendations included increased funding for SS benefits, it glaringly lacked a healthcare initiative. President Johnson wouldn't accept that bone again thrown to him, and after two more such unsuccessful urgings by the committee to augment SS benefits without healthcare, they made a U-turn. Johnson's persistence paid dividends. On September 2, 1964, the Medicare proposal as an amendment came to a vote and passed in the Senate. America had its first real health plan coverage for a large segment of its people.

On January 7, 1965, President Johnson's first legislation to the eighty-ninth Congress detailed a program including added hospital insurance for the elderly and needy children, all within the Social Security Administration. By this time, Social Security was so well entrenched in American life that tinkering with it was no longer considered a risk for any politician. Neither party would dare threaten SS.

Then came the usual debates and floor fights between the House and Senate versions of the Social Security add-ons. Introduced in March 1965 was the Mills bill, so named after another Wilbur, this time Ways and Means Chairman Wilbur D. Mills (D-AK), who got it out of committee and brought it to a final vote, with an unprecedented package for healthcare benefits.

In July, President Johnson sat in an office set up in Independence, Missouri, the home of former president Harry S. Truman, and signed into law the final draft. Truman became the program's first enrollee, and although its natural parents, Arthur J. Altmeyer and Frances Perkins, were standing behind him only in spirit, President Johnson, in his finest hour to date, started out with the well-deserved boast that older Americans finally have healthcare benefits. When Franklin Roosevelt signed the Social Security Act, President Johnson said that it, "was a cornerstone in a structure being built, but is by no means complete." How right LBJ was.

What has happened since is an integral part of the struggle not only to protect Medicare and its counterpart, Medicaid, but also to expand the coverage to match and perhaps even exceed that in other industrialized nations. Its chronology makes up an almanac of its own.

Federal matching programs were organized in 1966 with the feds paying up to 85 percent of the costs. That year also saw the selection of thirty-two private insurers under Blue Cross and sixteen other commercial insurance carriers to take over the administrative functions of the voluntary Medicare agency. By the end of '66, for a copay of three dollars a month, every American sixty-five and over was Medicare-hospital covered, and even the three bucks could be added to the public assistance checks if need be.

President Johnson didn't stop there. Before the decade of the 1960s was over and he left office, choosing not to run for another term in the heat of the Vietnam War controversies, all sorts of benefits were added to Medicare, though there were many people who still slipped through the cracks. After all, this was a new experience, and the Washington machinery was sometimes slow to respond. But Johnson had several watchdog agencies barking at the first sign of a leak, and benefits were increased accordingly. LBJ's last budget submission in 1969 included a 10 percent increase for Medicare. President Richard M. Nixon followed suit. Nixon added Supplemental Security Income (SSI) to the program. This added needed benefits for the disabled of any age.

Refinements to the Program

In 1977, on President Jimmy Carter's watch, the Healthcare Financing Administration (HCFA) was formed to separate Medicare and Medicaid from the Social Security Agency. HCFA became a multi-part agency that encompassed pediatric and pharmaceutical programs in addition to Medicare and Medicaid. President Ronald Reagan in 1982 called for the states to have full responsibility for the Aid to Families with Dependent Children (AFDC) and food stamps, but with the feds retaining full Medicaid control.

Finally, the Clinton years saw the most sweeping changes in Medicare law since its inception. William Jefferson Clinton signed HR 2015, the Balanced Budget Act of 1997 (BBA) that assured the program through 2010, reduced the rate of increase in payments to the providers, and added Medicare+Choice that allowed Medicare subscribers to add more coverage to their plans. The BBA also created the State Children's Health Insurance Program (CHIP), which is designed to assist those working families whose incomes do not qualify them for Medicaid, yet still do not enable them to afford private health insurance.

Before Clinton left office in 2001, he signed into law the Balanced Budget Refinement Act (BBRA) that made many changes in the total program. Its announced purpose was to soften the impact of payment reductions to providers of the BBA and stabilize the CHIP program. Other provisions in the HCFA programs were touched up, in attempts to provide some aid to those who were disabled but had returned to the work place, and also for women's care initiatives.

What all this has meant to the American people, when filtered down to actual implementation and benefits, may be another story, just another shift of the lounge chairs on the deck of the Titanic. Many myths surround the Medicare program and how extensive its present coverage. It still has many shortfalls, and, although an adequate stepping stone on the way to total coverage, it is certainly not the end all, nor what the country deserves and desperately needs.

Medicare's Machinery

Moving ahead to today, Medicare, with an over $300 billion budget, provides but a semblance of healthcare to our senior citizens and those with disabilities. And keep in mind it does not at this time cover all prescription drugs, hearing aids, dental care, eye glasses, or full nursing home care—the kinds of things disproportionately needed by senior citizens. Nor does it cover routine annual physical exams in any cost-effective way to allow hospitals and physicians to encourage their patient population to come in for such check-ups. Remember the old Ben Franklinism? "An ounce of prevention is worth a pound of cure." It surely isn't applied in this country in the twenty-first century.

Hospital clinics, in fact, routinely instruct their doctors to avoid using the billing index code for preventive check-ups on the forms for seniors that are sent to Medicare. Instead, they prefer that a diagnostic or procedural index code be used. This collusion is the only way the institutions find to circumvent the parsimonious practice of the HCFA.

As we will see, many physicians are becoming increasingly creative in trying to manipulate the billing forms in order to get their patients more coverage. And one more thing: It is definitely not free. There are fees and patient deductibles attached. Moreover, many U.S. physicians do not participate. It is certainly not obligatory. Physicians are permitted to opt out of the program. As time goes on, more and more clinicians—feeling the pinch of mounting overhead that includes the egregious soaring malpractice insurance premiums—choose to avoid Medicare patients. They cry poverty and insist that the bureaucracy involved in the filing of claims just makes the program cost-ineffective. "I'd rather see those patients as a courtesy—saves my office an awful lot of work for just a few pennies," is often heard said by many a clinician.

The present plan has two parts. Part A is for hospital incurrence; Part B covers clinical or doctor care. Included are: persons over sixty-five, eligible for Social Security or railroad worker benefits; the spouse of someone so eligible; those who have been receiving Social Security disability benefits for at least the prior twenty-four months; those with end-stage renal disease; and those with so-called Lou Gehrig's disease.

You would qualify, in essence, if you are over sixty-five, are a U.S. citizen, and purchase at least Part B of the plan. Part A is considered free of any additional fees to those who have paid sufficiently into Social Security or Railroad Retirement during their working lifetimes. If you do not meet the federal enrollment requirements, you may join up for a monthly premium determined by the amount of time you have paid into Social Security or Railroad Retirement. That premium at last reading was at an average of $175 per month. We will see how the Bush II 2006 proposed changes negatively affect all this.

Part B has a monthly premium attached that is the same for all enrollees. Today's $78 monthly price tag is usually deducted directly out of the Social Security payment. Part B helps cover physician fees, rehabilitation therapy services, outpatient hospital, and ambulance services. There are various coverages for rehabilitation equipment and disability needs, but they are usually judged on an individual basis.

So, although it is labeled total and complete medical coverage, it is neither total nor complete. At this time, Part B does not allow for prescription drugs, and how this will change after Part D's inception in 2006 if all sorts of manipulations planned by the Bush Administration go into effect, remains to be seen. Let's examine it.

Medicare and Pharmaceuticals

Prescription drugs play a larger role in the management of conditions of the elderly than all patients overall. In the general population, more of the diagnoses arrived at by doctors are treated with expectant care, and often no medication agents are needed. "Take two aspirin and call me in the morning" is a euphemism that has been successful in many cases. But with seniors, as the aging process alone adds to their woes, more times medications are required.

The most frequently seen geriatric conditions—diabetes, hypertension, and various cardiac/vascular syndromes—need more than two aspirin and a next morning's call. They take real drugs, often very costly ones. The gross profits made by the pharmaceuticals piled too high to hide. Something had to be done to quiet down the people.

Controversial Medicare Part D was taken off the drawing board and put into operation. It got underway in 2006. Its privatization rules and regulations are so apparent that many are starting to think this may be the first real step into privatizing the whole Medicare program. Part D is actually a successor to the failed drug discount card program several years ago that managed to attract barely 15 percent of those eligible.

Part D is not like the other parts of Medicare but was actually designed as a copy of the commercial insurance medication coverage plans. Parts A and B pay the designated fees directly to the hospitals, nursing facilities, and clinicians. But, in Part D, the feds remit to some 260 private insurance carriers. Then they in turn dole out to the pharmacy wings of the HMOs. They are then supposedly obligated to provide the meds to enrollees or the pharmacies.

There is also a pressure for Medicare enrollees to sign up, because holding off will potentially be expensive. There is only one opportunity to enroll without additional cost. Now. Electing not to pay into the Medicare drug plan and instead going out on your own to find needed medications, perhaps on the Internet or from Canada and elsewhere, could get you into trouble. You don't want to chance that route will dry up or suddenly become illegal. If so, and then you elect to join Part D, you are penalized 1 percent of the premium for the time you opted to hold off. May 15, 2006, was set as the day to jump on the Part D bandwagon without penalty. Seniors are perplexed, trying to decipher the system. The premiums are expected to average $35 per month. Be mindful. These costs are being passed on to our senior citizens, most with fixed incomes that might even go down, depending on where their savings lie.

There are also lapses in the program that stop coverage when the total layout reaches about $2,500 and then a doughnut hole kicks in again after $5,200. There are also deductibles that are preset for each drug.

Big Pharma was taking no chances. Their lobbies did their job. Written into Part D are provisions that enjoin Medicare from negotiating with the pharmaceuticals for lower prices on the drug products. Congress was just betting that good ol' American free enterprise competition would be enough of a control. Or so it was claimed. In that same token, generic imports from abroad are barred, using the claim that the agents would not likely be up to U.S. standards, even if from Canada.

It seems strange, even for him, that the Bush Administration calls Part D a gift to the Medicare members. Most of the estimated funded $720 billion will end up in the coffers of the HMO insurance and pharmaceuticals' treasuries. Its convolutions are so intricate that it almost forces enrollees to buy private insurance in which Medicare plays no role. That makes it even more of a perk for the HMOs than even Part A and/or Part B. The drug houses can pull out of the program if they desire (read: not enough profit). No wonder there is concern that Part D may fare no better than the aborted drug discount card plan.

A group of women at an old age nursing home gathered attentively around the sofa chair, where old Henry was holding court. His disheveled appearance and pot belly made him something of an enigma to attract such a crowd. Two attendants were off to the side and one asked, "How come old Henry gets all the ladies? Never could figure that out."

"Simple," said the other. "He is the only one here who understands Part D." ♦

Bills are being presented to Congressional committees that ostensibly would help clear up Part D. There are no timetables as yet for these revisions.

Medicare Part D does seem to be changing daily. Its marketing promises to be Big Business. With an eye on that $720 billion pot of gold, the almost hundred million dollars to be spent by the pharmaceuticals this first year on huckstering the various plans is well worth it. The HMO behemoths are going into business with the insurance guys to sell their drug plans through insurance company agents. Humana and State Farm are now hot and heavy into negotiations. Others are following suit.

The pharmaceutical industry in America, largely unbridled by the government, is running wild with the highest cost margins in any U.S. business. Due to expense that is growing every year, many Medicare enrollees never take their doctor-prescribed medications. It is as simple and tragic as that.

Iris Podenza, a widow for five years at age seventy-seven, was doing her best not to be a burden on her two sons and daughter, all of whom were struggling already to make ends meet in their own homes. All three were two-income families. There was no way they would make it any other way. I had followed her over the years for minor aches and pains, keeping her serious concerns like her diabetes and mild hypertension under control. But time was catching up. She faithfully came in for her semiannual exam but with a complaint of an annoying, relentless vaginal itch, pruritus in medical terms. My exam immediately told the story. Her occasionally erratic sugar levels had given rise to a marked vaginal fungal infection. Immediate attention was in order.

After the usual tests and back patting, I prescribed a daily local antibiotic and hormonal cream that would surely do the trick. That is why I was so surprised when she returned a month or so before her next planned visit, complaining bitterly of the pruritus. I reserved any decision until my exam. My look and palpation told me the condition had worsened. What was now a localized infection could easily metastasize and cause all sorts of systemic problems. Especially in a diabetic where infections like that become magnified and can be deadly. I was perplexed.

I had to nip this in the bud. Iris was a very aware and mindful patient. She always followed her doctors' orders.

"Iris," I started out, "how often are you using the cream?" I figured she was getting forgetful and therefore neglectful. That was not the case.

She looked toward the floor, awaiting my bawling out as she quietly admitted that she had used it barely once a week. She seemed to understand. "Iris, you know better than that. What is going on here?"

She took a deep breath, sighed, and pursed her lips. She said she just had no money that month to get all the salve I ordered. Next month, she assured me. "My budget ran out and I didn't want to go to the boys. They have quite enough on their shoulders this month. They don't need their old mama coming with her hand out."

Realizing what was happening, I went to the hallway closet, did some scrounging, and found enough of a sample supply of the meds, making sure the expiration date was valid. I wanted to cover Iris at least for the next month. I reminded her that unless she took it as ordered, she might as well do nothing. She nodded knowingly. ♦

The Iris Podenzas are not a rarity. They are created on a daily basis, when many Medicare patients need medications not covered by insurance or find they just can't come up with the tariff or any co-pays for the drugs that are "insured." And when many of the drugs have not yet concluded their seven-year period of being offered only as a patented, branded, and therefore costly product, less-costly generic options are not available.

Gaps in Medicare

Many seniors choose between food, the rent, and medications. Forget about a new Easter bonnet or an occasional movie and dinner at the local greasy spoon. And no one is anywhere near sure that there are any hidden helps in the forthcoming Bush II plan. In fact, the changes are so convoluted that it is making strange bedfellows all over again. The *Wall Street Journal* has come out against the Bush plan; the otherwise liberal and knowing Ted Kennedy had come out in favor. Go figure. Many an otherwise thinking and sensitive pol have sadly told their senior constituents that what we got is better than nothing and maybe, just maybe, it is a step in the right direction toward full coverage.

The counterproposal to the Bush debacle, the 2000 John Dingell, Jr., bill (D-MI), from the son of the late John Sr. of Wagner-Murray-Dingell fame, seems better in every aspect. I say "So what?" if it costs more, which it does. But the chances of that getting through the present Republican Congress are nil. There is considerable talk that the GOP version promoted by the president is so awful that in good conscience, it would not get by even a loyal Republican Congress.

Under the latest version of the Bush proposal, the conventional Medicare enrollees would qualify for two types of assistance. A discount card would be issued that could be used at all pharmacies; the exact allowances and for which drugs are not yet clearly defined. Then there is the so-called catastrophic coverage that is alleged to cover high-cost medications, but the parameters are, as yet, just as nebulous. A number somewhere between $4,500 and $6,000 a year has been suggested. Then there would be some added discounts for those who elect to use a fee-for-service plan. For many years now, Medicare officials have been encouraging their members to join those private plans. Privatization is still the ultimate goal of the president's proposals. Senator Edward Kennedy (D-MA) has already called it a "hoax...and forces seniors to join...(private carriers)...to get the drug benefit they deserve."

At best, the GOP/Bush "reform" covers only 22 percent of all prescription drug expenditures. In addition to paying out the difference, our senior citizens can expect to pay a $259 deductible, certainly prohibitive for many that may have been living on fixed incomes for years before the necessity of such treatments kicked in. Then there is a 20 percent coinsurance up to $1,000 and a 50 percent coinsurance for the next $1,000. That represents an outlay of at least $35 a month.

There is more, and it gets worse. There is a so-called "doughnut" with a big hole in the middle, leaving many Medicare enrollees laying out between $4,500 and $5,400 yearly for the medications that are not covered. The hole represents a period of time between when the minimum layout is reached and when the next level of coverage begins. That is where and when many of the patients just forego their medications and chance it, hoping that they will "make it" until coverage kicks in again. As many a media pundit has noted, don't even ask how or why that hole got there. You don't want to know. To those in "need and bleed," as they say, the hole can appear as wide and deep as the Milky Way.

As the vernacular goes, if you bother to read any number of explanations by the Bush Administration of its proposed Medicare changes, you will come away with any number of interpretations, and then some. That there are much turmoil and dispute within the president's own party is testimony enough of the controversy over this issue. As has been expressed by many a Congressperson, there is great concern by those who are facing reelection campaigns as to how they will explain this downgrading of Medicare.

For openers, we start with the BBRA, intended to stem the tide of reductions of fees to those physicians who were threatening to abandon Medicare in their offices, legitimately crying that the permitted fees just did not cover expenses. Despite the Bill Clinton statutes that were designed to ease the burden of reductions in fees, decreases were written into the law, with about 5 percent applied to each year through 2005.

On the other side of the coin, there have been some indications that with the advent of new fangled hi-tech equipment, especially for diagnosis, it has become impossible for doctors to keep up with the latest in technology without a modicum of increase in their fees across the board. Washington finally responded to that reality in April 2005 and announced that there would be a 15-percent increase in selected office visit fees to allow for those new expenses. However, although Congress rescinded a proposed cut in Medicare physician fees for the following year, a 4.3 percent trimming is slated for next year and as much as 26 percent total through 2011.

Not All Doctors Are Equal

The various specialties are treated differently, and almost as expected, those that cater particularly to the elderly were and are harder hit than others. For example, ophthalmology, a specialty that falls in that category, was earmarked for a nearly one-half slash in doctor benefits. Worse off still than these general ophthalmology practitioners were the specialists, and there are plenty of them—physicians who had long ago chosen an area of expertise within the field.

Literally overnight, these doctors found the payment for vital procedures, such as cataract treatments, say, slashed even further, without warning, and usually upon receipt of a letter in the mail. But their overheads and malpractice premiums continued to advance and even soar with alarming regularity.

Other specialties felt a similar sting. Family doctors and internists, especially but not only confined to working-class catchment neighborhoods, rely more heavily on a Medicaid and Medicare practice. They cannot possibly deny their over-sixty-five patients their Medicare coverage. But it seems ludicrous to those clinicians that although their expenses go up regularly, their fees go the other way.

And there are the specialties of geriatrics and physical therapy, by definition almost exclusively for the Medicare-aged population. Incomes for physicians in these fields are especially stressed, unable to keep up with the ever-growing expenditures.

By 2000, many a loyal patient would come back to their doctors for care or a checkup to suddenly find those offices closed to them for their lack of insurance coverage. The abandonment had started. "No longer accepting Medicare" is posted in more and more waiting rooms. Rather than toy with accepting Medicare as partial payment and the rest out of pocket from the patients to cover the difference (a questionable and possibly illicit transaction that many patients would reluctantly agree to in order to keep their long-standing doctors), office administrators find it easier and more fiscally sound just to refuse Medicare altogether.

Playing into this, too, is the potential threat of an audit by the HCFA, the shuddering thought of receiving yet another letter, perhaps this time explaining that after some nosing around, it's been found that the doctor is at risk for fines and charges, having been deemed a rule breaker. This despite finding themselves at odds with the HCFA while trying to serve their patients, repeatedly running into various rules and regulations that prevent optimal care.

And the boom lowers. HCFA comes knocking on the door. It is almost like receiving an audit notice from the IRS. "Medicare is just not worth it," is heard over and over again at the doctors' lunch tables. Medicare patients are refused. That is a doctor's privilege under the present law. The patients and physicians both lose.

Abandonment is putting it mildly. "Shameful and reckless" should modify the "abandonment." But, on the other hand, who can blame the physician, when expenses cannot be met? "Medicare is almost charity care," is how one doctor put it. Many clinicians are now limiting their patient clientele to exclude the over-sixty-five, and some even start the weed-out process at sixty, knowing that in five years, those patients will require the same treatments but then at fees that do not sustain the practice.

Sign in a doctor's office: No longer accepting Medicare patients. Or any patients who might be on Medicare someday. ♦

Then there is the proclivity towards limiting service to include a certain percentage of Medicare patients and drawing the line when others come for help. In one way, this makes the doctor seem altruistic and sensitive for even keeping some Medicare patients, and he is probably indeed doing the best that he can. But he is warning his patients, as painful as it is, that the handwriting is on the wall.

Office postings encourage the patients to write to their representatives in Washington, to describe their desperation. Not that the federal guys up on the Hill don't know what is coming down. But in numbers there is strength. Letters should be written. It is still the squeaky joint that gets the oil.

A very busy California orthopedic surgeon had replaced a knee for his patient years ago. Their long-standing relationship was mutually rewarding. When time came around for the other knee to need the same surgery, as predicted, he had to refuse care because of Medicare cuts. "It broke my heart, as a doctor and healer, to limit access to my care. These are patients who sent me pound cakes for Christmas because they were delighted with my attention and skill. But what can you do? The answer is the same for me as for the patients. And worth doing. Get angry. Write to your Congress person. In unity there is strength." ♦

The healthcare situation is but a reflection of society. The habits and practices learned over time are carried over. Doctors have all been taught that in a fee-for-service medical practice system, we can open and close our shops when we want, take a vacation when we please, knock off for an afternoon or weekend. Of course there are the acknowledged responsibilities, by law and ethics, when you qualify for and accept a license to practice medicine. But there are many forks in the road that can be taken.

One of the most serious of those routines takes advantage of the aforementioned major deficit of the present Medicare system—that it is not obligatory on the part of physicians to join up and provide care. That abandonment is permissible no matter the numbers. As a result, many communities across the nation, well staffed with doctors, have just a bare minimum or none at all that will serve the over-sixty-five population. Worse, this is the group who, because of age and infirmities, has little access to adequate transportation to regions where a clinician may be available. And that does not even address the emergency calls that occur frequently. Not all communities in the country have hospitals, settling instead for police emergency and ambulance services that can get you to a neighboring town that might be many miles away. There doesn't have to be multiple incidents. Just one tragedy as a result of absent coverage is enough to condemn the system.

The bottom line is that the physicians' bottom lines are continually the target of Medicare's administrators. But the medical community, while not all that quiet and yielding, is also not that proactive in its own defense, either. It is still steeped in the traditions from "back then," when militancy and organized protests were "beneath" them. Mass marches and rallies at various state capitals have been arranged from time to time, and doctors have been known to hire lobbyists to tweak the ear of the legislature. What with some members of Congress, including those in high office, being physicians themselves who entered the world of politics, optimism about having a "friend up on the Hill" has crept into doctors' attitudes. It remains to be seen how sympathetic an ear there is for the listening.

Part of the problem is that there have been so many contradictory directives and position papers issued to the public and the medical organizations that, as one local medical society spokesperson said, "You don't know whom to believe anymore. Or what."

Adding to the confusion are those same medical societies, who, as another excuse for not participating in their own salvation, have expressed concern over their members appearing personally greedy or self-serving when lobbying for higher fees. They avoid conflict with the many who are still holding an image of the physician driving around in a fancy luxury sedan and wearing hand-tailored suits, certainly not in need of financial sympathy.

Perhaps such discomfort stems in part from the ambiguous relationships between Medicare fee schedules and the private HMOs. They will adopt the same guidelines for fees as Medicare implements, but only when it is to their fiscal advantage. They might conveniently match Medicare when Medicare goes up, but they surely won't do the same when it goes down. This capricious behavior is the old pick and choose. Thus, Medicare policy has implications that extend well beyond its nearly 41 million beneficiaries.

The patients are also at risk. If Medicare decides to raise the physicians' fees, or at least not cut them, the people see what's coming—a raise in premiums.

Under federal law, premiums are set each year to cover about 25 percent of the total projected Medicare funding under Part B. The projected spending for Medicare Part B for the last two years caused the patient premium to increase by 34 percent. It took 34 percent more out of the consumer's pocket to cover that 25-percent allowance. In the future, this number will go even higher.

Medicare Life Rafts

Does Medicare need help? You bettcha. The Bush team and just about every media pundit are seemingly preoccupied with Social Security and what the Administration is planning for us before it leaves Washington. Independent observers, including those in the Government Accounting Office (GAO), have reported to the White House that the Social Security "emergency" has already been correctly labeled a bold-faced lie, in the genre of those weapons of mass destruction (WMD) that we were supposed to find in Iraq. The plight of the Medicare budget is serious and real. So it got some Oval Office attention, and another cut was put on the table.

The relationship between the federal government and the individual states has also been open to serious question. Every time state healthcare offices learn of a new Washington Medicare change, they wonder if the other shoe will drop. For example, when the 2005 Medicare revisions were passed in Washington to go into effect in 2006, kickbacks were written into the statute calling for states to return unused portions, what is mounting up to billions of dollars, so that the money can be used to pay for prescription drugs for the elderly. It is Peter robbing Paul, and another shift in the lounge chairs on the Titanic's deck.

Washington lobbyists are busy at work trying to convince Congress that the states will benefit significantly from whatever changes they propose. That helped get some wavering Congresspeople to go along with the president, not yet having been told about the funds that will be returned to DC coffers. State governments are starting to manipulate their spending practices to make it appear that the monies are being spent on other services, even Medicaid, rather than have to account to Washington for their Medicare expenditures and have to "claw back" all that the feds want. If an applicant is entitled to both Medicare and Medicaid, the states are enrolling them in the latter, not yet under the Oval Office's same spell. But don't hold your breath.

"It sets a dangerous precedent," said one governor. "Uncle Sam puts money in one pocket while picking another."

AARP

Small doctor groups and county medical societies are not standing alone in the battle against the Bush Administration's handling of the healthcare programs. The nation's leading association for the elderly, and the largest lobbying group in the nation, the American Association of Retired People (AARP) got some pretty heavy flack in 2003 when the Bush people announced their Medicare changes. The AARP had yielded to the insurance carriers and drug suppliers and issued a curious position statement that went as far as congratulating the president for his policy. The phones rang off the hook at AARP headquarters with messages of protest and member resignations. It now seems to be trying to rectify that gaffe.

Then, as the egregious policy of the GOP leadership ordered in obvious acquiescence to the pharmaceutical industry that less costly drugs from Canada be banned from import, the AARP drew the line. As the budget committees are starting their negotiations, AARP seems to be geared up for its own reversal of position.

The Senate in 2005 did stay its own healthcare spending slashes, to the tune of nearly $15 billion, by a crossover of a half dozen Republican votes, seemingly attributable to the strong demand by AARP that it pass. The Senate is now lining up on both sides of that coming struggle. From no cuts at all to the whole nine yards, battle lines are being drawn. The public is standing by, praying that the powerhouse AARP stays focused.

AARP did take a stand against the proposals the White House and the GOP advisors presented for the start of the privatization of Social Security. The clamor is that the Association will pick up their battle against the Medicare and Medicaid cuts, as well.

No one is daring to offer a prediction as to which way it will go this year. Legislators are all trying to come up with a number (read: how much to slash) they can live with and still face the voters. On one side are the president and his inner circle who insist "common sense reforms...ought to be adopted." The other side of the coin is obvious—that in this day and age, how can anyone possibly think of cutting healthcare funds? It is an insensitivity that is unbearable. The reality is that any and all healthcare programs deserve sizeable augmentations; yet, the GOP has our Congress merely fighting over how much to cut and expecting to play the hero if the cuts are minimized.

And the latest? As written, Medicare is anything but a real national health service, even for its limited enrollees. And more—it is, as noted, anything but "free." Those who are "entitled" pay two ways—once through their taxes into the federal treasury and then again at the "box office."

The gross Bush II Administration smoke and mirrors that were their 2004 Medicare campaign plans left us with added expenses and gaps in coverage. Co-pays and premiums took the hit. The money for Iraq has to come from somewhere. It is now coming directly from the backs of the nation's poor and elderly on fixed incomes.

In September 2005, basic Medicare Part D premiums were increased 13 percent. Across the board. Thirteen percent! Awesome and usury. That means that the present $78 per month will become $88.50 plus an added $35 average monthly outlay for that prescription drug so-called perk (read: for the drug companies). Fees are expected to jump yearly to cover inflationary increases and the pharmaceuticals' ever growing demands for more profit.

And lest we forget, the new Bush II Medicare statutes specifically prevent the HCFA from negotiating with the drug houses for any bargains based on volume—or public need. Nor do they allow it to purchase those less expensive Canadian or other foreign generics.

Do the math. That means that $120 per month will be taken from Social Security checks of senior citizens whose incomes will remain just about the same. The excuses fly. HCFA says the docs are charging more and need more for fancier care and those high falutin' tests. And more frequent patient visits.

Au contraire. The HCFA claims it is for new research, new technology, and the diabetes and cancer screenings encouraged by Washington, DC. All performed by private labs and medical supply manufacturers, for a healthy profit, of course. That $88.50 premium for 2006 was that $78 last year. $66 in 2004 and $58 in 2003. All on fixed-income seniors!

Medicare spokespersons claim that many patients are overusing the system. Big deal! They may very well be doing so, but why? Because of our basic insecurities that we are a nation without healthcare coverage. Because Medicare, always on someone's drawing board for extinction, makes the enrollees uneasy. Perhaps they feel they have to take advantage of whatever coverage they've got. Who knows what tomorrow will bring?

That is the key to this whole argument. With a true and stable National Health Service, we will be giving our people the assurance that care will always be available and free. Then they will use it wisely and learn anew.

Medicare in Our Future

The 2004 John Conyers (D-MI) healthcare bill HR 676 is one of several proposals floating around committees and is closest to reaching the floor for a vote. It is a decent start, to say the very least. It is indeed a *single-payer* statute, meaning that only one federal agency would be responsible for all accounts receivable and payable. A reduction in bureaucracy is dramatic and welcome. While it does start us toward a federal-government-controlled, universal, and comprehensive national healthcare system, it does not entirely eliminate privatization. So it is time for the people of the nation to rise up and do even better.

Maybe we should start by asking not where Medicare is heading but where it is being taken. Next we must ask, how are we going to improve it, maintain it, guard it, and protect its future? Remember, this is our health we are talking about. While we are standing about, debating the issue of healthcare, people are not standing about, idly waiting for something to happen. They are getting sick and dying. Neither death nor illness takes a holiday. What we need, we need now.

The overall view of the state of Medicare is precarious. If there were one word to describe the plan the Bush Administration has for Medicare, it is "privatization." And if there were three letters to summarize that privatization as an acronym, try HMO, Health Maintenance Organization, the machinery that is being proffered to America as the solution to its healthcare needs.

Medicare is not the only program facing such a fate. There are Medicaid, Social Security, and the nation's public schools. All have been extensively examined. The Edison school system of privatization is already undergoing pilot programs in several areas of the country, and Medicaid is, in some instances, even further along than that. Some states have already instituted the means of total conversion of their Medicaid to privateers. On Social Security, the jury is still out and that debate is continuing.

There can be no further doubt. The Bush II White House set its sights on destroying Medicare as we know it. Along with the total alterations planned for Social Security, the dismantling of Medicare as a government-run healthcare program is first in the cross hairs of the Oval Office. The ploys of demonization that were so effective an era or two ago are being resurrected subliminally in attacking Medicare. "Socialized medicine" as the work of the Devil has been so successful that it has become almost a given. Now there are other slogans that are ballyhooed. "Compassionate conservatism," the catchwords of the first Bush II campaign in 2000; "choice," as though this were being borrowed from the abortion struggle; "reform," which appears to be a synonym for "improved." The changes being offered are beneficial to the insurance company-banking conglomerates and the pharmaceutical companies that were heavy donors to the Bush/GOP election campaigns.

The $100 million given to the GOP on these past two presidential hustings was twice that sent over to the Democrats. After all, the donors weren't burning all their bridges. They were just making a calculated guess, unless they knew something about Florida 2000 and Ohio 2004 that we didn't, then. Now it is too late.

American seniors were not considered a political force by the GOP, despite the power and membership of the AARP. The demonization of the 1930s was being counted on still, and the threat apparently worked. The major deficits facing the government in the coming years are often used as the excuse for having to cut benefits such as Medicare. The tax cuts tendered the wealthy, the cancellation of the estate tax, and other comforts for the comfortable are never mentioned.

But the sad events are unfolding as the Bush campaign agenda takes hold. When the gigantic HMO-privatization tsunami moves into place, Medicare will be no more. The profit margin under Medicare is just too low to continue to tolerate. Arthur Altmeyer, Frances Perkins, and Lyndon Johnson must be spinning in their respective graves.

Medicare HMOs

The move started in 2003 when the Senate Finance and the Ways and Means Committees in the House passed bills to shove Medicare closer to full privatization, warning that without drug benefits under federal Medicare, disaster loomed. They said a rectification was sorely needed. The median income for Medicare's 41 million members was at $14,500, and over 25 percent spent more than $100 monthly on needed medications.

But this is clearly a subterfuge. It does not take a total turnover of the Medicare system to arrange for medication allowance. The aim is total takeover of Medicare by the private insurers in America. With the flick of 51 percent of Congress, Part C could be added to cover all medications.

The lawmakers have a Part C plan of their own—to get the healthcare business out of government hands to put it where they think it belongs—in corporatized America, solely in the hands of private insurers and conglomerates.

The HMO and the less-controlled-by-the-private-insurance-industry Preferred Provider Organization (PPO) were considered passing fancies back in the 1980s when they were spotty throughout the country. Then, insurance carrier moguls hired groups of member clinicians for fee-for-service and paid either per patient treated or by capitation—a set fee for the entire member group on the carrier, whether group members sought care that month or not. After the Clintons, the president and wife Hillary, fostered the plan, it took off full steam in the early 1990s.

These HMO/PPO plans are great, depending on the beneficiaries. If you are old and sick, forget about it. FDR's cassandric statements, as LBJ remarked at the Medicare signing, are coming back to haunt. The enrollee pays in for Part B as noted, and, of course, when the federal monies are deemed insufficient (as will, of course, happen), the member has to cough up the difference.

Does anyone out there actually believe that a private system of healthcare delivery with a bottom line in mind and run by an insurance company instead of a medical practitioner will provide better healthcare to the needy? Can that be?

Just what has happened in the system at this early date in its transformation to an HMO-run unit? For openers, there is a word for that ,as well—dumping. That descriptive word says enough. If indeed there are those doctors who are still accepting Medicare patients for whatever reason, they are then often finding ways of referring the very ill and medically needy to the public healthcare sector.

Most private docs would much rather, of course, take care of the well patients who are there for preventive check-ups or who have long years of doing well on maintenance meds. For those other crises and obviously long-standing and enduring traumas and medical needs, the patient is simply sent over to a public institution, put into the category of a "teaching case," and house staffs take over.

HMOs are canceling their contracts with the HCFA. It is a frequent occurrence; in fact, rates of pullout are rising as we speak. For example, the Cigna Corporation, a major healthcare HMO-player, recently announced that it was discontinuing the coverage under Medicare for hundreds of thousands of enrollees in such banner states as New York, New Jersey, Connecticut, Delaware, Florida, Virginia, Maryland, and Texas. Aetna, another mega-HMO company, has announced more moderate plans for dis-enrollment, but there are daily hints and statements that it is a work in progress. It is not adding any seniors, that is for sure.

The American Association of Health Plans (AAHP), a trade association of the so-called managed care industry, has simply stated the operational priority for its members. Medicare payments are still not enough to adequately cover the costs of caring for the elderly, even with dumping. It added that as Medicare reimbursements were rising at a rate of 2 percent per annum, costs were rising from 10 to 12 percent per year. AAHP said the practitioners were being "forced" out of the program. The HCFA answered by saying the drop out rate was less than anticipated.

That means the HCFA knew it was going to happen, that the hemorrhage was going to increase, and it stood by as though healthcare and prescription drugs for the elderly were expendable.

The pronouncement that many drugs not covered by federal Medicare would be covered by the HMO Medicare is yet another deception. The Part D prescription drug plan with that doughnut hole and co-pays and the rest of that morass will still leave many seniors out on a proverbial limb.

In the mid-1990s, citizens flocked to their HMOs for the alleged extra benefits like dental and chiropractic and ophthalmology care and medications. The expected happened. Beneficiaries paid more each year of enrollment, with co-pays that were not affordable by people on fixed incomes.

Hospital benefits demanded a $100 copay, every day, from seniors who never see that kind of buck. But it was enough to persuade all too many Democrats to sign on with their vote, including Ted Kennedy and his Senate pals. Rating groups like unions and consumer activists are closely watching the California experience.

Washington continues to debate with both sides fighting for what seems like the same end but perhaps from different motives. The Democrats want to adjust more chairs on the deck of the Titanic, with different co-pays and a smaller hole; Republicans argue for more HMO membership so they can move faster down the path to full privatization. They both seemed to back off last year, neither party wanting to send their candidates back on the campaign trail trying to explain to their audiences why they will have to do with less and more expensive medical care.

An old man finally succumbed to his mortality and was greeted at the Pearly Gates by St. Peter. "You have to choose which one you want," Pete informed his new comer. "Heaven or Hell." When the gentleman immediately opted for Heaven, he was told it was available, but to choose only after inspecting both. Then make a final and irrevocable choice for eternity.

The man had to acquiesce and took the elevator down to Hades, as a formality to the new rule. But there he saw great weather, chaise longues, libraries, a buffet table piled high with gourmet foods, music, and servants to cater to his every whim. Puzzled, he took the elevator up to Heaven, where he saw clouds, angels with harps strumming welcome tunes, hors d'oeuvres, and the sun up above.

He returned to base camp and told St. Peter he had surprisingly selected Hell, fully understanding the decision as final.

He hopped into the down elevator cab, and it opened below into a blizzard of ice and snow, filth everywhere, stale food, and dirty water. "Wait a minute," he told the Devil. "When I was here for the inspection, it was beautiful and different."

"Ah," said Satan, "that was before *you voted."* ♦

Bush Administration Proposals

Many a pundit and columnist have complained that the proposed Bush plan is so convoluted and duplicitous it almost seems deliberately calculated to confuse the voter in Congress and in the country to accept it out of desperation and hope for the best. The debate over Medicare was that whenever enrollees signed up for whatever plan, they were locked in for a year. HCFA rules do not assure that drug coverage would be complete or that co-pays would not become exorbitant.

Medicare beneficiaries face a large increase in the years to come. The HCFA has stated that increased costs have forced this action. On the other hand, it was also declared that Medicare payments to doctors would be slashed (and were) in 2004. President Bush underscored this treachery and signed legislation to increase Medicare spending for doctors' services by over $54 billion during the next decade. AMA president Yank D. Coble, Jr., said the Medicare formula for doctor payment is severely flawed.

The denouement is that word again—privatization. The drive toward universal healthcare started in the first Administration of Franklin Roosevelt with the genius of Arthur Altmeyer and Frances Perkins that finally got off the ground in the Johnson Administration of the mid-1960s has been in the cross hairs of every Republican Administration since, and there was no respite from the Democrats in between. It was another case of silence indicating acceptance.

Bush II's second State of the Union Address on January 28, 2005, included the announcement that Medicare was one of his goals for "reform." He used that catchword for the first time. He added that he wanted our senior citizens to have a "choice" and a plan that provides prescription drugs. But then insisted that privatization was the only way to go. It was naturally interpreted that the 86 percent of those who were in the federal program would have to join the 14 percent who were already HMO Medicare members. Just like the public school and Social Security presentations by administration spokespersons, the obfuscation can be cut with a knife. But it all filtered down to one dictum—to get drug coverage would require HMO membership.

Robert Hayes, president of the Medicare Rights Center, called the Bush proposal a "cruel hoax." But the Bush Administration legerdemains continue to this day. The various Oval Office statements and then those by his spokespersons at press conferences and from the floor of Congress are so twisted, some Republican Congresspeople are even wondering out loud if the president understands what he is saying, or if he grasps the problem of the increasing numbers of seniors and the decreasing services for them.

Geography also is playing a role. The senators from rural states where HMOs are rare are breaking with the White House, urging that all Medicare members get drug coverage and that there must be no coercion that forces the seniors to take a private plan, either for the drugs or because of higher rates on the federal side of the coin.

Because of this two-tier system, it appears as though traditional Medicare and HMO Medicare are competing against each other for enrollees. This is bizarre, in that the funds for both come from the same coffer—the federal treasury. However, because HMOs have more leeway than the traditional, they can find and use tricks to eliminate the more costly patients. Dumping is only one means. Layoffs, facility closures, and denials of various expensive medical services can be opted at will. Why the people prefer Medicare HMOs over Medicare remains a mystery.

Looking ahead, the Medicare debate over privatization will soon reach its peak. HR1, whose chief architect is William Thomas (R-CA), will fully privatize Medicare by the year 2010. Thomas has already boasted that HR1 will "end Medicare as we know it." There is good reason to believe that the 2004 "handouts" to Medicare members were election year hype. On the other hand, as each year goes by and as the number of seniors rises, there is more and more of a clamor that Medicare be that institution Lyndon Johnson said it would be—just the start of full healthcare service for everyone.

Bill Thomas is no stranger to the Medicare battle. Several years ago, he chaired a Congressionally established commission, along with Senator John Breaux (D-LA), who already had a record for trying to push Medicare financing solely onto the backs of senior citizens. Under their recommendations, the HCFA would issue vouchers to eligible seniors worth a magic 88 percent of the contrived average Medicare premiums. Whoever opted for any Medicare program and its included premium, the difference between the 88 percent and the actual premium would have to come out of their own pockets. These costs could sometimes be higher than HMO Medicare! The HMOs would be enrolling less-sick patients, passing the more needy onto traditional Medicare.

This would, as a matter of course, drive up the costs of the program, lead to higher premiums, and make that out-of-pocket copay too expensive for many. President Bill Clinton was not having any of it, despite its bipartisan imprimatur. The 2000 elections shelved it for what the newly elected Bush Administration sought—enlargement of the HMO programs, ultimately leading to full privatization.

How do we save Medicare, at least certainly until a better plan comes along and something like Conyer's HR 676 becomes law, so Medicare recipients get the benefits of total healthcare?

Obviously, for-profit HMO Medicare plans are not the answer. We do not need them practicing medicine without a license. Putting more MBAs and insurance carrier moguls in charge of our health only continues to put profits ahead of our well-being. That concept itself is deleterious to our health. Anything that stems from it would be, as well.

When the going gets tough, there then arises that old demonization cry of socialized medicine and the exclamation that financing such a program would take many more billions. The scare of increasing payroll taxes and dipping further into the federal treasury, making for a larger deficit, has people believing that we cannot afford total healthcare.

But the American people are paying into Medicare one way or another, and they are slowly but surely learning that the Medicare HMOs are squandering upwards of 25 percent of premiums on their awesome administrative overhead, advertising, executive salaries, and profits. Traditional Medicare has beautifully kept those same costs at a 3-percent level. Quite a difference. Hopefully, the people will not accept bailing out private Medicare HMOs as a form of corporate welfare.

Short of what we really need and deserve—a total and universal healthcare package for everyone—there are ways to fix the Medicare crisis now. Medication costs must be included in whatever Medicare is to become. The HCFA must have the power and even obligation to negotiate with the pharmaceutical companies for the lowest price possible for their members.

Using Canada as a paradigm would also be a good start to full service for our people. The threat of accepting less costly Canadian medications into our system must be real enough, so that U.S. drug houses fall into line. And Medicare's service must be an obligatory part and parcel of every American physician who takes that Hippocratic Oath to serve and accepts a license to practice the trade. Compromise and healthcare are not compatible concepts.

MEDICAID

Medicaid is the linchpin of the American healthcare system. It is the closest thing we have to a program for the general population. In terms of beneficiaries, it is certainly the largest health insurer in the country. Its 52-plus million enrollees top that of Medicare and, symbolically, that other 43 million who go without any coverage whatsoever.

In fiscal terms, its circa $165 billion budget represents about 13 percent of the total national healthcare expenditure. It was intended to cover the expenses of low-income people who were elderly, blind, disabled, on public assistance, or even among the working poor. Poor people with annual incomes of no more than $7,908 and a maximum of $3,950 in tangible assets qualify under the present rules. For a family of four, those numbers are $11,604 and $5,800.

Some of those criteria, as we will see, have changed dramatically since Medicaid's inception back in 1965 when its enactment was a part of President Johnson's Great Society. Medicare took top priority at the time, and Medicaid was largely a product of the House Ways and Means Committee. Representative Wilbur Mills (D-AK), its powerful chairman, worked along with that other Wilbur, Cohen, who later became Secretary of Health, Education, and Welfare.

It was an outspoken Rep. Mills who became more celebrated by his lone dissent on the Warren Commission when he voted for conspiracy in the Kennedy assassination. Mills' term was short-lived. His midnight dance around the fountain in Boston with companion Fanny Fox proved so embarrassing an escapade that he resigned his seat. There were Washington observers who suggested that his role as an iconoclast in pushing for Medicaid and then the dissension on the Warren Commission had marked him for extinction.

Medicaid became an integral part of the HCFA. The issue of its finances came into question. Congress made it clear that Medicare was a federal responsibility, while Medicaid was put under the aegis of both state and federal agencies. The shared role was based on a formula that counted the states' per capita income, although the federal contribution could never go below 50 percent or over 83 percent.

There were guidelines for eligibility established by the HCFA, but most were turned over to the states. Because most states only had a single working welfare agency, Medicaid was just tacked on. It seemed to make sense. But that lined it up with public assistance, and the seeds as a welfare program were sown from its onset. HCFA ended up with five branches, including Medicare and Medicaid, but because of the stigma attached to Medicaid as a welfare program, it became an HCFA stepchild. Congress and the Oval Office soon assumed that same attitude.

Half of Medicaid's enrollment is children (26 million), the rest divided between adults (12 million), the elderly (6 million), and the blind and disabled (8 million). Congress occasionally alters the eligibility criteria based on the number of pregnant women and their dependent children, as well as varying requirements that cover the disabled. But the variations remained small for the most part until the Ronald Reagan years, when there came stark changes.

Suddenly, the yardsticks were tied into whether the person was actually on the welfare rolls in that state, thus eliminating many of the working poor who had no chance of affording private or even HMO healthcare. Time limits were also put into place, depending on employment and efforts to stay off the unemployment and welfare queues.

It got complicated, and many people woke up to a mailing that cancelled their Medicaid coverage, even when there was a scheduled surgical procedure or current and pressing medical need. Medicaid offices were besieged by lines of people maneuvering to fight the system.

Medicaid Manipulations

As the Medicare fiasco took center stage, what with the Bush II Administration's loud efforts to seek its so-called reform, Medicaid took a back seat. And some of Medicaid's advantage over Medicare was obvious. Medicare has no drug allowances; Medicaid has some, but that is also changing. George W. is taking full aim at Medicaid. Watch out!

For openers, there was the "block grant" the president introduced. This meant that those formula-based federal funds would be sent to the states to be used for whatever programs the governors deem needy. Medicaid is not usually at the top of the pile. Even many of the state houses opposed this idea; it got too confusing and too burdensome on the local offices. When things would go awry, as they often did, the blame fell on the states, not the feds.

It gets more tortuous. New York, for example, does spend more on Medicaid than any other state, but look at the demographics. Booming, younger, urban populations require more substance abuse programs and pregnancy termination facilities (banned by federal law since the Reagan Administration), than other states. And more money to spend on the expanding older population's needs of expensive nursing homes and home care.

So, while the Kaiser Family Foundation analysis reveals that the state of New York covers more needs for more people, it also highlights the gap in allocation left by the percentage of the pie it receives from Washington. Ironically, the more you need, the bigger the deficit. That is when the federal formula is supposed to kick in.

When the states call the White House for more funding to maintain their programs, the answer is that you were already given a block of money. Spend it any way you deem necessary. It is like a parent giving the child a weekly allowance and when that extra lollipop is cried for, it is denied, and the papa feels that the absent treat is a great lesson in money management, a reminder to act wiser next time around. As many a headline has glared these past years: WHITE HOUSE TO STATE—DROP DEAD! The sad truth is that is exactly what happens. This is not a missing cherry sucker on a stick we are talking about. People die when they do not receive valid and adequate treatments. It is as simple as that.

The truth came to light as the 2005–2006 budget was revealed. The Administration has announced that there will be no more funding this year for health service programs. Some even had to be cut because the federal government did not tender the state treasury with cost of living increases. The answer to Reverend Jesse Jackson, Sr.'s, question still stands. "Where do we get the money for needed healthcare, etc.? From where we are squandering it!"

Seventy percent of Medicaid money is allotted to the elderly and disabled. When there are visible cutbacks, it is those who need it the most who feel the greatest pinch. Likewise, the race card is played hand after hand in the dealing of Medicaid. Health problems being what they are, by the very nature of our two-tier system, they are worse for minorities and people of color.

State reports shows this to be true. The poor develop more serious health problems and are less likely to have coverage that will get them optimal doctor and hospital care, and often it gives them none at all. Along with poor nutrition, endemic patterns, and faulty sanitation, that gap accounts for their shorter life spans than whites. It accounts for a lesser quality of life all around.

All men may have been created equal, as that axiom goes, but without clean toilet facilities, a well-balanced diet, and guaranteed healthcare, that par disappears the moment of birth, or sooner—during their mothers' gestations. In fact, the studies are clear on that, as well. The gap in the U5MRs of the country's different ethnic groups can be attributed to the quality and quantity of the prenatal care offered to our pregnant women. It is directly proportional, starting with white, privately-cared-for women; black, privately cared-for women; white and then black Medicaid-covered patients; and then those with neither coverage nor care.

In 2005, Ohio slashed 25,000 participants from its Medicaid rolls and took 15,000 more from their drug coverages. All budgetary issues. Tennessee won in its appeals fight to drop 323,000 from its expanded Medicaid program. Texas, President Bush's home state with a Republican state house, is at odds with the Oval Office because of the Bush plan to include Texas in his strategy to drop $60 billion in Medicaid money over the next decade. Almost 3 million of those 52 million Medicaid beneficiaries are Texans.

Where Is Medicaid Going?

What is in Medicaid's future, and how does it fit into the campaign to get a national health service for everyone in the country?

The answer reflects what is happening in our social order. Medicaid is just a part of that system. For while all these cuts have been going on, the Bush people have voted in a $290 billion tax break for the richest sliver of U.S. citizenry and is planning to make that a permanent law. The estate tax that was cut in 2001 is up for debate and is still not a closed issue.

More than half of the nation's bankruptcies are attributable to healthcare expenditures. And although declaring bankruptcy and putting yourself behind that eight ball of last resort is bad enough, it will get worse. The relief and forgiveness, the light at the end of the tunnel of financial ruin, the hope that there will be a better day, is being squelched by the Machiavellian GOP Administration bankruptcy statutes that went into effect in 2005.

Further punishment awaits those who dare to let down their credit card companies, unable to pay out the highest of interest rates that lay on top of their already exorbitant bills for medical care, and the financial hole goes deeper and deeper. There is no American dream for those who can only pay the monthly minimum.

It is apparent to all. Pro- and anti-administration media are saying it like it is. The lead editorial of the nation's paper of record, the *New York Times*, on March 12, 2005, read that Medicaid is in the line of fire. It described the critical service Medicaid was providing, with the message that Medicaid is already skimpy and that further cuts, or moreover, denial of increases in its allowances to keep up with the cost of living indices, would doom the program, maybe forever.

The failure of the Clinton Administration to propose and pass any semblance of a national health program in 1993 left us with our abysmal HMO system and Medicaid and Medicare programs that are always on the chopping block when budget considerations are being made. The saving of the sinking "Titanic" will take more than that shift in its deck chairs; it will demand a total commitment and a patching of its rupture. And it must be based on an admission that healthcare for the economically deprived is more strikingly absent than for any other part of our aging population.

Medicaid and Medicare are only pieces of the HCFA puzzle. There are those elusive medications and the special services and facilities for children that we need to think about, too. That the reimbursement allowances for both Medicaid and Medicare are just unrealistic within the U.S. market place. That there is simply little to no access to our most skilled and trained and experienced physicians. That Medicaid has been branded as a second-class citizen, and until it takes its place in the mainstream of American medicine, it will always remain the abused and threatened stepchild.

Neither program will get its just due until we start with the HCFA forest. Then the trees that are Medicare and Medicaid will be preserved and stand tall as the gateways to a true national health service.

CHAPTER 6

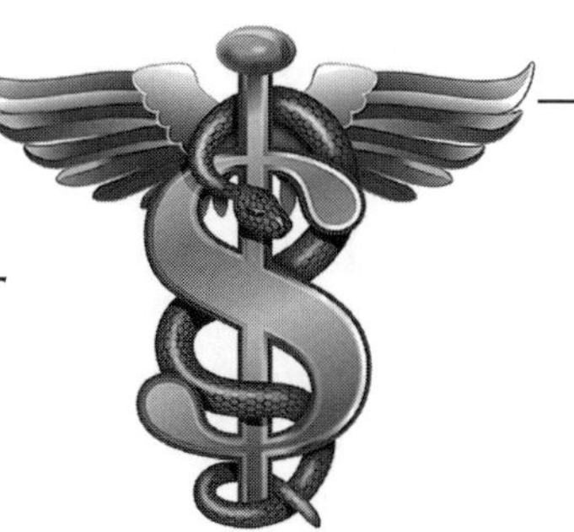

IF THE GODS MEANT FOR US TO BE HEALTHY, THEY'D HAVE LEFT THE DOCTORS IN CHARGE

It all happened so quickly; the nation's almost 900,000 physicians never knew what hit them. While they were keeping an eye on the specter of communism and its socialized medicine, those forces that saw an opportunity to take over an industry moved in the back door. Only now they are prancing up the front walk. Before you could repeat after me and recite the Hippocratic Oath, the banks and the insurance companies set up what we are calling, at their insistence, managed care. Mismanaged care is what it has become.

Privatization is becoming the rule of the day. In 2000, George W. Bush coined a new term, something he and his GOP think tanks are very good at. After all, on his first campaign, he told the people he was a "compassionate conservative," whatever that oxymoron means. For his second term, when he actually got a majority of the popular vote, he said he wanted Americans to be owners, owners of their own property, lives, and fate.

He picked up the gauntlet thrown down by every president before him in post-WWII America. Healthcare as a policy seemed to have been brought to the forefront on the 1992 hustings by then candidate Bill Clinton. President Clinton eventually shaped-up the Health Maintenance Organizations to a point of such refinement that today, better than two-thirds of all insured Americans are HMO members. And that number is climbing. The billions of dollars spent on healthcare have not diminished—not that they should. It is just that they have been shifted from doctors' accounts to insurance company coffers. The doctors were labeled providers, the patients became members, and a whole new gestalt of American medicine was born.

Let us lean back into history and see how it got this way. Instead of an MD, how did people with business school MBAs take over our healthcare? How in the world did they come to dictate the extent of any diagnostic workup, decide how long we would stay in the hospital post-op, or even decide if we were allowed to have the surgery in the first place? How did they get to monitor the labor and delivery of a pregnant woman in the obstetrical suite or audit doctors' patient track records with their many satisfied and well customers, and then insist on refunds from doctors because of an afterthought-determined excessive treatment?

Bertha Devin was an eighty-year-old woman, by chronology and appearance. She had been a part of our office setting for several years, having been followed after her bilateral mastectomies for breast cancer. She was seen regularly and was being closely regulated for her chemotherapy. The last visit, two months ago, was thankfully routine.

Bertha's hometown in Middle America knew her well. The local merchants and utility service people considered her a friend as well as a customer. The hospital felt the same way.

An oft-predicted crisis finally happened. Bellyaches and pains after supper. Her call sounded urgent indeed, and she was seen the next morning. An ultrasound picked up a series of small yet clinically significant gallstones, but the workup couldn't stop there. Bertha had built up some fluid in her abdominal cavity and a shadow suggested hydronephrosis, with fluid backing up into her left kidney. I ordered the radiology service to run off a CT scan but was summarily informed that in view of her already completed testing and the subsequent GB diagnosis established, there would be no CT clearance. Her primary doctor had to refuse. Test denied. None of us involved was happy with her kidney picture. A cause had not been confirmed.

The office arranged for her hospital admission a week later, and she underwent a successful cholycystectomy, stones and all. But a gynecologic surgeon who would accept Bertha for her Medicare coverage just could not be located in time. Bertha was overstaying her welcome as permitted by her Medicare HMO and was discharged, with plans to find a hospital and a consultant who would investigate her renal swelling and cause thereof. Stay tuned. Bertha is. ♦

The Birth and Death of a Healthcare System

Where did it actually all start? When did U.S. medicine become so unique in the developed world and establish such a resistance to any similarity with public programs, standing by as others borrowed a page from the U.S. Constitution and its Bill of Rights that became a paradigm for every republic that followed ours?

Congresses have been debating healthcare almost as a matter of routine since the nineteenth century. Early on, there was no real champion or national office candidate who made healthcare a linchpin to any campaign. Mother England rubbed its palms together with glee as the new world went through several decades of turmoil as the Colonies were feeling their growing pains. The U.S. became a bicoastal nation. They were trying to live up to their constitution, but no one talked about healthcare.

It was not until after the end of World War I of 1914–18 that healthcare was deemed a more pressing matter by each Congress. The Glitzy Age of the Roaring Twenties put us on some sort of a pedestal that had every malcontent in Europe and beyond wanting to come here and walk on "the streets that were paved with gold."

The Great Depression circa 1929 brought reality and us down to earth. We were fragile after all. The 1930s New Deal of FDR and its Social Security became the marvel of the whole world, and many a European political scholar wondered aloud how we had not gotten around to establishing that ever-elusive healthcare package. They all eventually beat us to it.

Then came the epoch that so many living Americans went through in person—the 1940s failure of Wagner-Murray-Dingell, the Fishbein/AMA demonization, and finally, the 1965 advent of Medicare and Medicaid. Those, along with some tack-ons, finally established at least our potential to have a national healthcare program.

There were some notable additions. The Richard Nixon Maternal-Infant Care (MIC) program in 1970 that halved maternal and perinatal mortality among the American poor within a year is among the proudest accomplishments in our history. But there was bad news, as well. No administration since RMN, gave the MIC its needed funding, and the Ronald Reagan crowd of the 1980s started its depletion toward its low point of today.

The Clinton Era

Move ahead to 1992 and the start of the Bill Clinton Administrations in Washington. Or should I say Clintons? That book is far from closed. How strong an influence or how high an office that former first lady and now Senator Hillary will assume in the years to come is the topic of conversation on every lip in every back smoke-filled room in the nation's capital.

The Hillary Rodham imprint on healthcare started from the moment husband William Jefferson took to that first presidential campaign trail in 1992 and made his mark in U.S. history. There is even historical evidence that it was the topic of conversation and strategy more than we were led to believe.

In May 1993, coalitions and activist groups gathered to protest our lack of a national healthcare plan. But their picket lines did not pace in front of some government office, hospital, or insurance carrier headquarters. Instead, they amassed in front of the New York Times building in New York, symbolically protesting the media's "rationing of healthcare news!" There had been a New York City council's 12-2 vote urging Congress to put our national healthcare on its agenda that went unreported in the *Times*.

The print media were not the only outlets at fault or the only targets of the organized protests. Letters to the editors and TV talk show hosts came in by the thousands. Demonstration lines were formed and flyers distributed that clamored for the electronic media to "get with it."

A Congressional committee had already been assigned a March 1993 bill, "The American Health Security Act," signed on by fifty-eight members, but it never got out to the U.S. listeners or readers. It was modeled after the Canadian system as a federally sponsored single-payer plan that included every U.S. physician and eliminated co-pays and deductibles. But it was essentially ignored by the print and electronic media. Within these pages is most likely the very first time most readers have ever heard of such a thing.

Poll after poll that reported most Americans' favoring such a movement went unheralded, as well. There were endorsements by labor unions, including those with their own existing types of coverage, and such reputable journals as *The Atlanta Journal-Constitution* and the *St. Louis Post-Dispatch*. Most of the push in the papers and the six o'clock news came out for Bill and Hillary's competitive managed care plans.

One would have believed from the conservative Republican and Democratic think tanks and their appurtenances that the "Jackson Hole" guys, the group of managed care do-gooders that convened in Wyoming to discuss our futures, were doing a good job for us. As it turned out, they were doing a number on us.

It is surely no coincidence that the Clinton Administration was feeling its oats, gleeful at its certain success in passing the North American Free Trade Act (NAFTA) that was to go into effect with Canada and Mexico in January 1994. As the corporatization of America was moving into high gear, the Clinton loop was marching hand-in-hand with the national conglomerates all the way. A federal national single-payer health plan was the last thing it needed. Surely it would stand in the way of its proposal for "managed care."

A small backlash ensued. The "Harry and Louise" ads were about to break on network TV. "Harry" and "Louise" looked just like us on our living room couches, sort of a take off from the Norman Rockwell images a few eras back. After a laymen's description of the managed care system that was putting the initials HMO into our lexicon, Louise would lament, "There must be a better way."

As political writer Norman Solomon described, we were starting to see the two faces of the future senator from New York. When Hillary Rodham Clinton finally met with the Jackson Hole Group, her mission moved into a higher gear and approached the final stages. After all, in the White House was a president who had campaigned strongly on the needs for America to have a proper healthcare plan worthy of our great nation. So coming out of the Wyoming retreat with something, anything, would be looked upon as an accomplishment and a fulfillment of that campaign promise. Never mind that they stuck it to us.

In that Jackson Hole lodge, presidential emissary Hillary Rodham Clinton met with quite a clan. There were reps from the insurance industry, bankers, and administrators of lobbying institutions that were in the Oval Office favor. They all really believed and lived by the lessons of GM Charlie Wilson that what was "good for General Motors was good for America." But in glaring absence were those labor leaders, consumers, and front-line medical professionals who worked in the trenches. Solomon's "Big Five" of the insurance world—Aetna,

Metropolitan Life, Prudential, Cigna, and Travelers—formed the Alliance for Managed Competition, totally in line with the Clinton aspirations. The HMOs were their common links, with all of their already heavy investments.

Both Hillary and the Democratic Party countered the "Harry and Louise" ads with those of their own, promoting the Clinton viewpoints. "We want our system back," demanded First Lady and spokeswoman Hillary, as though she were in agreement with Harry and Louise. Nobody asked, "What system? Back to where?"

The Health Insurance Association of America (HIAA), a trade organization that represents the small to medium-sized insurance companies was revealed to be the perpetrator of the Harry and Louise promos. Big surprise! As they sat by and watched the major insurance houses gobble up the lesser lights and narrow the field of which ones would write healthcare policy, those smaller insurance carriers had to be afraid their number was up. It was as though Sherman antitrust, that 1890s classical Congressional statute that was the first to control monopoly formation, never existed.

An actual conspiracy had been put into motion. The insurance industry was invigorated by the Jackson Hole soft and hard sells that had convinced the president's spouse and trusted partner. The print media started to call on them to take over, parading that consolidation as an advancement and selling it to the American public. "Single-payer" became the battle cry, as long as each of the insurance companies was potentially that single-payer and not the federal government. Morris Fishbein and the demonized socialized medicine were very much alive.

Healthcare became so limited and narrow that, almost as though it were after a handshake deal, certain carriers backed down and paved the way for a dwindling few to stay in the healthcare delivery business. The "Big Five" took over, and there were and are continued rumors, based on back room negotiations, that one of them will swallow all the others.

And if "single-payer" became the battle cry, the Jackson Hole "white paper" became the rifle and the HMO the bayonet. It had all the right words—health and maintenance. It was as though some nebulous entity was being created that would generously provide healthcare for the people of the USA. The plan and hope was to have the folks talk about their HMOs as they talked about their Norman Rockwell family doctors. Even with the same affection.

Enter Managed Care

As America inched closer to accepting managed care as the only option available to us, the power structure that was aligned with the insurance/HMO promoters decided they had to cross every "t" and dot every "i." They were taking no chances. They wanted an insurance policy of their own, and world events were their impetus.

Washington and its State Department were flush from what was conceived as a victory over "Godless communism." The Soviet Union had fallen under the weight of the relentless Cold War, the arms race, the space adventures, and, finally, the cooperation of the Soviet hierarchy. Mikhail Gorbachev, soon to be the ex-Soviet premier, took President Ronald Reagan's advice and "took down that wall" in Berlin. Germany was once again unified, something that Joseph Stalin pledged would never happen as long as there was a USSR. He was not wrong. The Soviet Union ceased to exist.

"Free enterprise" had taken over the Soviet economy, Marx's specter was no longer a European threat, and the United States was indeed the world's only superpower. Ignoring that there were and are still very visible pockets of various forms of socialism in the world, from little Cuba to humongous China, managed care purveyors reverted back to what had worked an era before—the demonization ploy that was "socialized medicine." It had always been lurking, although subdued.

Cuba was dismissed by its size and containment under the harsh boot of the U.S. blockade and China by the Western propaganda machine constantly turning out item after item about how it was moving ahead only because it was adopting Western-style commercial capitalistic practices. Historians seemed to forget that in the first years of the 1917 Russian revolution, Lenin had instituted the New Economic Policy (NEP), designed to get much-needed funds to build what he conceived as "socialism." The world is watching and waiting as the Chinese picture unfolds.

The Canadian and English Models

Another scapegoat that would serve as a demon had to be found, and it was. Articles kept appearing in the establishment press about how the two most heralded federal healthcare systems in the world were failing their people. Canada and the United Kingdom were looked upon with scorn.

We were told of the delays of weeks and months for the people in those Second World nations to get their needed surgery, cardiac pacemakers, renal dialysis, and just about all other medical procedures. We started to hear and read about and were led to believe that Canadian and English physicians did not meet the caliber of their U.S. counterparts, although nothing was further from the truth. A comparison and analysis of healthcare in Canada and Great Britain, manipulated by U.S. politicians and the HMO managed care promoters, was the fodder for the next phase of the conspiracy.

In the era before the need for demonization, English, Scottish, and Irish medical schools were looked upon as the finest. Along with the reverence of Oxford and Cambridge as educational meccas, many medical training facilities in the UK had been praised with a touch of jealousy as being at the top of the didactic heap. Dublin was held up as the model for obstetric practice. London- and Edinburgh-trained surgeons were viewed with awe.

National Health Services (NHS) seemed to have changed all that. Hospitals and doctors were suddenly offering inferior treatment to the English people and their neighbors. Scores of Brits and Scots, men and women with means, were now flocking to U.S. medical centers to get it done the American way—by a private practitioner working under fee-for-service. The truth lies elsewhere.

We have been led to believe that Canadian hospitals are now second rate compared to our own and that Canadian physicians are suddenly poorly trained and honed. While it is certainly true that one must always take into consideration the sizes and cosmopolitan make-ups of the nations involved when deciding "best in show," Canada is not to be looked down upon. By every medical parameter, Canada compares favorably to the U.S.

Canada is consistently in the five best every year for its U5MR. Even white America's is a shade below Canada's. Perinatal mortality, maternal mortality, and neonatal mortality, the original standards used to measure a nation's health, have the U.S. lagging behind. Life spans for both sexes are three years longer in Canada. And, most significant, while Canada spends about 9 percent of its GDP and the USA spends a whopping 15 plus percent on its healthcare, the USA still has almost 45 million without coverage and over 40 million more considered to have inadequate care. There is not a single Canadian without full coverage.

When former vice-president Al Gore sought a medical/surgical center to operate on his seriously brain-damaged son, he chose a renowned Toronto pediatric neurosurgical team. He chose wisely. The operation was a success. ♦

Every country's citizens reap even more benefits when healthcare is a given, a right, and, therefore, a non-issue. Having a comprehensive healthcare program frees up businesses and employers to deal with other employee benefits and gives the potential workers a better, less desperate place from which to negotiate their terms. That remains one of the bugaboos in the States.

Whereas President Reagan instituted his further restrictions that curtailed Medicaid coverage for many, based on a two-year grace period and tied into welfare roles, the Canadian system has neither a time limit nor an association with public assistance. In the U.S., there are many who avoid low-paying jobs for fear that they will earn just enough to disqualify them from Medicaid enrollment, yet nowhere near enough to afford any semblance of decent healthcare coverage.

In Canada, that does not come into play. Workers take on some of the less rewarding jobs, even temporarily, because there is no fear or threat that their coverage for themselves or their families will be cancelled, curtailed, or limited in any way.

Another upshot of a universal system is the reduced labor costs at the factory level. Catastrophic medical expenses occurring from serious on-the-job accidents, generally the largest component of any settlement, are rare in Canada, common in the USA. That is only because all Canadian citizens are guaranteed that basic and very adequate repair and rehab.

Even product liability (PL) costs are affected. From those Canadian manufacturers that export to the States, their PL premiums are as much as one-third higher than pure domestic producers, as protection against potential lawsuits stemming from product failure possibly incurring medical expenses not covered in the USA

In expanding its operations just recently, Detroit's General Motors clearly stated that the reason for opening an assembly plant just across the border in Ontario was the savings of almost $1,600 per auto, budgeted for its healthcare package for its work force, unnecessary in Canada with its federal program.

A *World Business* report notes the real issue is that the average American worker can expect up to 10.85 percent of his/her wages to be deducted for worker's compensation. That is twice the Canadian average. This is only because worker's compensation plans in Canada are federally run; in the States, they are a maze of private and public systems at all levels of government. And with profits attached that are always protected by law, the costs soar.

There is a bleak future if this type of disparity continues and enlarges. As our population ages and life spans grow longer, Canadian businesses will be able to out-compete their U.S. counterparts because U.S. medical expenses will outpace general economic growth. That head bone and toe bone are still connected.

Those corporations with both Canadian and U.S. operations run their businesses with different systems on opposite sides of an international border, even though their business vantage point is the same. They obviously see and take advantage of their Canadian annexes in hiring workers, knowing the Canadians' healthcare is protected by law and therefore, not a corporate expense. How and why is it, then, that the corporations remain so opposed to a similar plan in the USA?

Those corporate execs are running scared. They are each a member of the same club, and they all have the same ambitions and concerns. Their respective bottom lines. Knowing that healthcare is the third largest single segment of the U.S. economy, they dare not leave their fold and support a government takeover of an industry that is at least 15 percent of our economy. Therefore, they actually run counter to their best interests because of what Presidents Calvin Coolidge and George W. Bush have clamored for—ownership America. Keep the government out of our lives. Let free enterprise reign. No interference from above. You know the rest.

The United Kingdom story is similar. England boasts as fine a U5MR as the rest of the Western G-7 countries and has improved steadily since the inception of its National Health Service (NHS). Reports from Britain are almost predictable.

Great Britain is going through trials and tribulations that might be expected in the U.S. after a national health service gets underway. It will have to endure constant bombardment from its opponents and those "ownership"-oriented politicians.

But, the NHS in the United Kingdom has been the saving grace of all their people, if only because of the peace of mind it brings them. The worry about outpatient procedures, major surgery, and intense and prolonged hospitalizations that are the fear of every American (save the very wealthy) just no longer enters the thinking in the British Isles. And that, despite the shortcomings of the system. Remember that at last reading, over half of American bankruptcies were because of healthcare burdens.

The NHS is not entirely free. There are able-bodied and under retirement late middle-agers who copay a part of prescription medications. Those reported shortages of hospital beds, operating room time, and hospital personnel, though wildly exaggerated, are not without foundation. Not entirely. Certain allowable operations are delayed for an "excessive" time due to a lack of surgeons and operating room facilities and personnel.

There is certainly, exactly like in the USA, a distinct shortage of nurses. The shortage has been traced to the low wage scale that has driven many from the profession and prevented others from entering it. Some hospital centers have been forced to close their nursing schools for lack of interest and enrollment. Just like the U.S., the UK has been trying to recruit nurses from abroad, notably from the Third World, who will take a lesser wage and consider it a boon as compared to their own economies. Trade unions are peeking through the nursing back doors, and the rightwing media moguls are getting ready for the attack, always chomping at the bit to proclaim that the fault lies in the NHS system.

Patients who wrestle, for however long, with a decision to have a certain procedure often cry out "excessive" when they come to grips with it and decide to go ahead, want it done yesterday. Any sort of a delay, heretofore acceptable, becomes deplorable and abusive. Mind you, this only pertains to so-called elective operations. What has to get done does. Hippocrates' law rules in the UK as in the U.S.

Without question, the great problem about this form of socialized medicine is not in its concept and its functioning in principle, but in its funding. When and if there have been waiting lines for surgical procedures, if there is an insufficient number of hospitals, or if there is not enough professional staff, it is due to a failure of the government to allocate the needed funds to correct the problems. It is as simple as that.

The nursing crisis happening in the UK and echoed in the U.S. is a case in point and a microcosm of what is happening elsewhere in the medical industry. And for the exact same reasons, with an identical solution.

The U.S. Pentagon spends more in minutes than what is needed to solve each and every major healthcare problem facing our nation in a year.

A change in priorities is what it takes. Like I said, it's the money, stupid. The Margaret Thatcher and Tony Blair years have not been kind to the British NHS. The known shortages of personnel and facilities are related without question to a constant drain in PM budgets that have robbed the system, leaving it underfunded. Restore the pounds sterling, stupid.

The Canadian model has also been shown to be suffering from a steady drain on its original budget. There is more and more talk in Canada that its acclaimed NHS will be reverted to the provinces, with appropriate federal funding slashes. If that trend continues, Canadian services must suffer, as well. Restore the dollars, stupid.

Worth asking, logically, is if adequate funding is possible. Answer: of course it is. It is in England and in the United States, as well. Where are we going to get the bucks? Always the same answer: from where they are going! From out of the pockets of the insurance and banking moguls to go into the hospital and medical services needed to serve the people.

We Gotta Start Somewhere

Rep. John Conyers (D-MI) put it as succinctly as possible. The principal author of HR 676, the United States National Health Insurance Act (USNHI) that would establish a federally sponsored single-payer healthcare, said his bill would free our nation "from having to put up with the outrageous costs that keep millions...from receiving medical care and needed medications."

HR 676, although not a fully funded, tax-supported program but instead still relying somewhat on individual premiums (albeit small compared to a privately enrolled HMO managed care system), does address the pitfalls that are gripping the Canadian and British systems—money. HR 676 has several built-in safeguards against future gutting.

But Conyers and his pals are in for a long and tough haul. Instead, there is more shifting of the Titanic deck chairs being planned.

Paul Ellwood, MD, an HMO pioneer who founded the first Jackson Hole group back in 1971, is back into the fray after a several year hiatus spent recovering from a serious horseback riding accident. He watched as Hillary Rodham Clinton endorsed the Wyoming statements that left us with managed care, which never got past committee in Congress, and then fell to ex-Speaker Newt Gingrich (R-GA) after the GOP sweep took over Congress in 1994. The Gingrich Contract with America (read: more of the same) took healthcare reform off the Congressional agenda. His mephitic departure from the government a year later did not restore its place on the docket. Doctor Ellwood, now back in good health, has indicated he plans to reconvene the Jackson Hole group and its agenda. But to what end?

Ellwood has expressed bitterness over the Clinton failure to enact any sort of a plan and has hubristically said the group needs to include physicians and healthcare professionals. But still no mention of labor leaders, from health unions or otherwise, consumers, or in-the-trenches victims of the system.

Overheard in the OR as the surgical team was about to make the patient's incision: "Let's make it snappy. His insurance only covers a two-hour operation." ♦

Incrementalism

One of the greatest dangers facing the movement to get national healthcare underway is that of incrementalism. As each of the states and even some cities have become more and more frustrated without a decent healthcare plan, they are encouraged to resort to working out a local program of their own. But that falls right into the hands of Big Pharma, the HMO conglomerates, and the Washington honchos who are carrying out their bidding.

The pitfalls are numerous. Nepotism, cronyism, and payola in all forms are bad enough at the federal level. Imagine how rampant they can get when there are no independent overseers that could possibly guard against such practices at local levels. States and major cities simply do not have the trained personnel and the administrative means to construct and carry out such a massive and delicate undertaking as providing something so vital as healthcare for its people.

It is bad enough when crookery is discovered in general construction, plumbing inspection, or highway and bridge building, for example. People are put at risk when a faulty roof crumbles or leaks, a roadway collapses with the first frost, or sinks and toilets fail to provide potable water or don't flush. Imagine, then, ailing people being denied doctors, nurses, emergency rooms, and other vital medical supplies and facilities at that moment of need.

Nevertheless, states have made noises that they are considering such plans of their own.

The various states that are now in control of the Medicaid programs financed from Washington are all vying for those funds. And they are constantly lobbying for more. As noted, there are concerns that the state-level bureaucrats might be too far out of the public eye, despite their geographical proximity. Without enough scrutiny, there rises a greater chance for misallocation, resulting in denial of medical services in favor of spending on other programs preferred by the state houses.

New Jersey, even prior to the new 2006 Corzine Administration, had started a health awareness program for its 78,000 state workers as a means of alerting the public to what is in store for them.

Tennessee's state government has announced that there has to be a "disenrolling" of nearly a quarter of the state's 1.3 million residents who are now covered by either conventional Medicaid or the HMO/Medicaid programs.

California, still smarting under the Proposition 13 budget restrictions a generation ago, is starting to impose a cap on enrollments in state healthcare programs, despite Governor Arnold Schwarzenegger's campaign promises otherwise. With its Kaiser HMO leading the way, California, and even Ohio, Minnesota, and Texas (the home state of President George W. Bush and the highest number of the uninsured in the country), have all sounded off in trying to effectuate some form of healthcare plan for those without. None have come up with the formula, and always for the same reasons—funds, personnel, facilities, and a general proper bureaucracy.

Michigan officials have announced a plan of their own after receiving some vague grants from Washington for close to $2 million. It remains to be seen what they will do when that is used up—likely after the first day of operation.

Governor Kathleen Sebelius of Kansas has also put out some form of plan that involves small businesses in an attempt to cover Kansans who now go without.

Maryland has made rumbles directly aimed at forcing Wal-Mart, that world's largest private employer, to offer affordable employee healthcare coverage, now glaringly absent. Wal-Mart has mobilized their legal staffs to start compromises with Annapolis.

Oregon, the state that announced several years ago that it had formulated a plan, is starting to leak at the seams. In 2005, five Oregon hospitals accused the state house of breaking their brokered agreements for payments, and suits have been filed for recovery. That means, of course, that bureaucratic costs go up, up, up.

Illinois, back in 1999, decided to start from scratch. Named for a popular Archbishop, the Cardinal Joseph Bernardin amendment was put on the Illinois ballot and received 83 percent of the voters' approval that declared healthcare a basic right of every Illini. With that showing, tens of state senators signed on as sponsors of committed legislation with the hope of pushing along a state healthcare referendum. We are all watching and waiting.

Montana, with the highest percentage population of any state without any coverage at all, is wrestling with new options to alleviate the problem. It seems that the state legislatures are redoing all of its programs for the poor. Food stamps, welfare checks, and medical care will be affected if its House goes forward with a proposal to cut funding for all of those programs for the needy.

Pennsylvania, New Hampshire, and a host of other states are gearing up, with committees being formed in their state legislatures, as those cuts from Washington are expected.

Believe it or not, New Hampshire's august body of lawmakers is considering a rider to the present statutes that will require some forms of co-payments even from those families without any reported income at all!

About half of the 700,000 Medicaid enrollees in Kentucky will be paying at least two dollars more for each brand-name prescription drug as a result of budget pinching.

New Mexico's legislature is readying a debate on how much can be slashed from the state's Medicaid budget in order to comply with federal guidelines so that maximum matching funds are delivered.

Vermont is following suit.

West Virginia is undergoing a total Medicaid restructuring, the budget being kept in mind. The recipients in the state would receive only the services they "need" and have to show up for medical appointments under a new program aimed at cutting costs.

How's this for chair shifting of Titanic proportions? North Carolina state authorities noted that one-fifth of their residents go without health insurance. Layoffs and job attrition increase those numbers daily. The Raleigh assembly met to seek out funds to cover this segment of the population and, facing impending cuts in Medicaid expected over the next decade, NC has its job cut out for it.

Considered one of the leading people-sensitive states in the South, NC is also working on a plan for thousands of the state's medically uninsurable to buy coverage from a pool that now covers high-risk coastal homeowners. Number one, the protection would have to be bought; number two, it would cover only 10,000 of the estimated 1.4 million now without medical insurance safety nets. The bill's proponents add, with a straight face, that it would be a saving to the state because those uninsured would no longer come into the state's medical system as emergency patients after trauma and disasters.

Massachusetts Republican Governor Milton Romney has now made headlines as he suspiciously starts his run for the White House in 2008. He publicly expressed his concerns about providing some sort of coverage for the state's 700,000 uninsured. In the spring of 2006, he signed legislation that made it mandatory for all baystaters to enroll in some sort of healthcare plan. The governor's program included vetoes for certain demands that the employers had to lay out for what the private carriers set for as a premium. The governor also insisted, in no uncertain terms, that the federal government had no place in any plans for healthcare delivery and that the days of single-payer are over.

The ink of his signature wasn't dry before critics of the plan exposed its folly. They pointed out that about twenty years before, Governor Michael Dukakis, before his presidential run, also celebrated what he called a major healthcare breakthrough, only to have it implode before two years were up.

As reported by Harvard medical school faculty staffers, Doctors Steffie Woolhandler and David Himmelstein, it is a sham from the get go. The Romney bill expands Medicaid coverage, anything but valid in view of Washington's planned funding cuts over the next ten years. It offers subsidies for low-income people, and then those making more than three times the declared poverty income would have to buy coverage or, and get this, pay a fine. Yes, the bill actually states that if you do not buy what you cannot afford, you will be penalized! I need your imagination again to figure out how a family living on the edge and usually with two jobs will come up with the thousands now required by law.

Massachusetts is notoriously always at the top of the cost-of-living states. The private carriers and pharmaceuticals are frothing at the mouth waiting for this windfall. There are other provisions that involve businesses of certain sizes to get state subsidies to provide care for their employees.

Woolhandler and Himmelstein finished their discussion with a single statement that says it all. "The legislation offers empty promises and ignores real and popular solutions." They were referring, of course, to a federal single-payer plan. Political watchers are waiting to see what mileage Governor Romney gets out of all this furor when he goes on the presidential campaign trail in a couple of years.

A New Dictionary of Neoterms

But, with the advent of the HMO, doctors' power and prestige are waning, their independence eroded to the point where what they tried to avoid back in the twentieth century, being considered a tradesperson, has become the reality. Worse, they are employees of the HMO unit and are reminded of it every day. There is now a new language that dramatizes the new order. Doctors are now called "providers" by the HMO, and those who were once called patients are now labeled "clients."

The family doc made a house call in the early evening to an ailing teenager. After the exam, he issued and explained a prescription. Then he asked to use the lavatory. Tucking his bag by the grips and putting on his overcoat, he mentioned to the parents that he had noticed a loose handle on the toilet and he used one of his pocket medical clamps to tighten a bracket screw. As he was halfway out the door, the dad said, "Doc, I wonder if you might take a look at a drip in the kitchen faucet. Your rates are cheaper than the plumber's." ♦

Those doctor and patient sobriquets are an unofficial vernacular now in use. There is now a set of official terminology that has been put into the medical lexicon, and likely, future editions of medical dictionaries will have to include them to be complete and up-to-date.

Co-payments are the portion of the bill the patients must kick in. The amount is set by the HMO and is not negotiable. They are often a small percentage of whatever fee rate was set by the HMO, also not negotiable.

Out-of-network doctors have either been rejected by the HMO or have themselves refused membership for any number of reasons—usually simply resistance to accept what they consider too low a remuneration. Forfeiting automatic referrals, these clinicians can instead charge whatever they like over and above the copay, assuming they can attract and keep those patients willing to pay. Some physicians have refused any HMO membership, relying on out-of-network patients or those who are not HMO clients. That type of doctor is slowly but surely disappearing.

Out-of-pocket maximum is an annual limit on spending that is found in just about all health insurance policies. Medications and other aids and out-of-network doctors' fees often go toward reaching that number, and, once patients spend that money, they pay no more.

As a result, clinicians, justifiably concerned that the medical office will not get reimbursed, hesitate to embark upon the exhaustive and unwieldy paperwork to ensure payment. They shy away from performing even the simplest of tests in their offices that, until now, were convenient and even commonplace and often give immediately treatable diagnoses; basic urinalyses, pregnancy tests, or screening urine cultures can allow for on-the-spot treatment. Instead, the process is delayed until the commercial labs provide the information. Offices that have their own service labs are fading away for non-coverage.

Balanced billing refers to the practice in which doctors and hospitals bill directly for care provided and charge patients over what the HMO allows. This practice is denied in Medicare and some HMO plans and is allowed only in the out-of-network setup. Many policies will not count this against the out-of-pocket maximum.

Diagnostic Related Groups (DRG), cynically known by doctors as Decreasing Reimbursement Guarantees, are now applied by Medicare and many HMOs. This is a system whereby a diagnosis for any and every condition has a set fee for both the hospital, if involved, and the clinician. The gradations of that particular pathology are not taken into consideration as individual but only as a lumped-together group.

For example, and any condition can be used, suppose one patient has a severe cardiac crisis that demands intensive care/therapy, the extensive use of facilities, and even life supports for a significant length of time. Another patient with similar symptoms is tendered the same admitting diagnosis but is stabilized and recovers in just a day or so after a minimum of care. Since the two cases had the same admitting diagnosis, regardless of the care and outcome, Medicare or the HMO will reimburse the hospital and doctor the same amount.

It has been determined that the times when lesser or more intense care are needed will even out in the end; as time goes by and more clients are seen by the provider, the numbers will dilute the differences. The DRG allowance is based on what will happen over a course of time. To show how the DRG system has been PR sold, many a physician has even praised it.

Dumping then becomes a common practice and is an offshoot of the DRG system. It has become, shamefully, a rather common practice when the admitting attending physicians, and even the house staff, transfer the more demanding case to another hospital, with creative reasons why this is necessary.

Or else, depending on the quality of the HMO insurance, they will tell the ambulance to keep on going to a public hospital emergency room, where the patients can never be refused. Except for an occasional case that tweaks the intellectual interest of the attending-in-charge or the resident physician for teaching purposes, dumping is applied.

There is, however, a universal ethical and even legal practice that states that abandonment of a patient is never acceptable. Physicians, for whatever reason, cannot ever simply withhold treatment in one form or another. Assuming the patient is reasonably stable, not in a life or death mode, and able to travel with or without an accompaniment, the doctor must triage with that in mind.

If the doctor feels unqualified to handle the patient's situation, a referral to an appropriate specialist is obligatory, without exception. This must, by all medical ethics, include assuring that the patient and accompaniment have written documentation of the referral physician's name, address, and contact phone number. The doctor must also place a call or be in direct contact with the specialist to alert the next service of the reason for the transfer and be assured the patient is expected and will be accepted for care. This can be as simple as a reference to a public institution and a house or paid staff on duty. The same rules apply. I cannot imagine a more vicious break with the Oath of Hippocrates than abandonment.

To show how established this practice is in medicine, even if the doctor is denying the patient care out of principle, morals, or religion (such as in a patient who, for example, has requested a legal termination of a pregnancy and the doctor's religious principle says otherwise), that physician must send the patient somewhere for counseling or management. Total abandonment is not an option.

Gatekeeper(s) is the correct term and intended meaning for what they do. These are hired hands of the HMO/insurance carrier that guard the gate, or entry to the hospital, or the call for more intensive care that requires permission by the HMO for the doctor to proceed with treatment.

The gatekeeper is often a registered nurse with a physician overseer. This was exactly the case with my Jessica Riggins (Chapter 1). This doctor, usually semi- or fully retired from his/her own practice, is now in the proverbial driver's seat, deciding if a patient is going to be permitted to have certain medical procedures or hospital admission. The gatekeeper is given a summary of the client's (read: patient) history and physical exam findings of the referring doctor and renders a decision from a desk many miles away from the patient/client and doctor/provider, never setting eyes or hands on potential admitees. The decision is proffered and considered final.

I wonder what Hippocrates would say about that. Hands-on was a significant part of the Hippocratic Oath.

Carve outs are what every hospital and physician fight to avoid. They both hate to hear those words. If the doctor defies the gatekeeper and the HMO, and the hospital is somehow convinced, infrequently, that the patient is to be allowed an inpatient stay, or if the patient remains in the hospital as an inpatient over and above the time allowed by the HMO, the insurance carrier will "carve out" the days and medical fees as a deduction from any reimbursement.

The hospital will bill the patient for an overage on the HMO allowance, and the patient/client is responsible legally...unless. Unless the doctor/provider and patient/client raise a fuss and make waves (which will sometimes work out, à la Jessica Riggins), the billing stands. Sometimes it does not matter how loud the protest.

There has been many an occasion when, years later, the HMO carriers will audit their member doctors and decide that too much has been paid out, due either to an error in the procedure translation or a mistake in the original approval for treatment. The HMO then invoices the doctor/provider, sending a statement for payback of what may be years of service and hundreds of patients/clients.

If the doctor/provider resists and refuses to honor this bill, the HMO can use legal collection means or simply deduct that amount from future earnings. It goes without saying that the medical office in question could be dismissed from the HMO service rolls. The HMOs always come out ahead.

Capping is the method of payment that the HMOs are using to entice doctors to join up. Here, the HMO assigns a catchment area of potential patients to that physician's office and pays in, sometimes monthly and sometimes annually, a set fee regardless of an office visit having taken place. Actuaries claim that, by sheer numbers over the years, the reimbursement will average out as adequate as compared to a fee-for-service rate.

Just think about that. This means that the clinicians will be paid whether or not they see the patients! There are already thousands of incidents where patients have been managed over the phone or starkly dismissed. "Take two aspirin and call me in the morning," has thus been taken to a new extreme.

This is especially significant when the clinician and the HMO are working under a for-profit system and where that motive is up front and always a factor.

Tiered plans, where the co-pays are adjusted according to the deal made, are used by some HMOs when it is deemed that the negotiations with their providers did not go that favorably. For example, if the HMO decides that a particular physician or hospital/clinic has a more costly service, the copay could be passed on to the insured individual to make up the difference.

This is a good selling point to the employer, who, told of this arrangement, finds the plan more fiscally inviting. UnitedHealthGroup and others started a pilot project over the objections of their customers who voiced opposition to plans that required them to change physicians to avoid higher copays.

COBRA

COBRA, the Consolidated Omnibus Budget Reconciliation Act, is as aptly named as anything that has come down the pike. It is a true snake in the grass. COBRA allegedly gives workers and their families who lose whatever health benefits for whatever reason the right to continue policy rewards exactly as they always were, for a defined period of time, deemed adequate to either pay up or find other coverage.

No one has yet explained how this is to anyone's advantage except the insurance carrier that gets to keep the client for a fee that, exorbitant to begin with when the breadwinner(s) was getting a wage, is now fully unmanageable. Try to pay the premium when you have lost your job.

Any of life's events can qualify you for a COBRA policy: divorce, layoff, transition between career choices, reduction in working hours that would disqualify you, etc. The only possible perk for the ex-employee or ex-anything is if there were a pre-existing condition that could invalidate the worker for any new coverage or translate into a premium that would be considered usury. A COBRA policy must be offered. You just have to come up with the dough.

One of the myths of COBRA, and one way that it has been sold to an unsuspecting public as a great deal, is the rationalization that because the premium had been based on a wholesale policy sold to many employees, it must have been a bargain. But many a laid-off worker has discovered that with a little legwork and maybe Internet surfing, a less costly policy with the same benefits or better can be found.

Debunking the myth further, in many instances, a mass sale of a coverage plan to a group comes with a higher cost. The thinking is, and likely true based on actuaries, that the larger the pool of clients the greater the chance there will be those with more severe ailments, and thus the whole of the group must pay for the most costly individuals. It is like the rotten apple theory. The one with the worm makes the whole barrel smell bad.

I was covered for my near fifty years in practice, said one retiring pediatrician. It was through my own medical society, and I figured I had been paying the best rate for the best care. But then, when I was no longer eligible through the society, I decided to use that same plan on my own as a COBRA supplement, and I had an awakening. I could have bought that same coverage all those years, either a singular policy or as a Medicare additive, for far less. It was then that I learned that a premium had been charged for all those colleagues who were not in such good health. ♦

There are a few other catches to the COBRA plan. For instance, if the employer goes bankrupt or just closes up and goes out of business and the company plan that covered the worker is no longer in existence, a COBRA policy is not always available. This is why many a worker has found out that shopping around or using a policy of a working spouse will get them better benefits for less. The ex-worker then realizes that for those many years, the deductions from the salary check and the cost of any follow-up COBRA were certainly no bargain. Of course, there are no such things as refunds from any said overpayment.

HIPAA

HIPAA (Health Insurance Portability and Accountability Act) is one of the latest arms added to the HCFA. It was born in 1996 as part of COBRA, allegedly to protect workers' privacy when they either changed or left their jobs so that healthcare coverage was continued—at a cost to be determined, like COBRA, often beyond their means. It reached the physician and public eye in 2003 when the accountability portion took front and center. Physicians were instructed that there would be penalties extracted if it were discovered that patients' records, either office or hospital-generated, were exposed without tacit patient permission.

It was almost amusing to sit in on a HIPAA orientation lecture given at hospital conferences as the staff was being instructed to do what had been done since Hippocrates—protect patient confidentiality. All obviously stemming from the rapidly growing changeover to electronic records and data keeping from the conventional paper charts, Title II of HIPAA was suddenly announced as going to be enforced in 2005.

There surfaced a seemingly valid concern that electronic data would be available to anyone with a computer and some basic electronic skills. Among its selling points was that lawyers, unfriendly family members with an array of motivations, investigators of all sorts, and especially insurance carriers who were looking for pre-existing conditions to render the prospective client ineligible for coverage, would be able to gain access to such private information. It became jocular practice at hospital staff meets for a physician describing a certain patient's case to stop in the middle of a sentence for fear of violating HIPAA regulations.

Wait. There is more. The HIPAA act as written in Congress specifically allows for the patient's existing or potential HMOs to access the chart information, a la Jessica Riggins, as a means of further controlling patient care. There are several rather intricate exceptions written into the laws that govern HIPAA. Different carriers have negotiated with the authorities and struck up their own deals as to how often and under what circumstances they are entitled to patient records. It is as if they were exempt from the law.

Come to think of it, they are.

I knew it was time to quit when I had a term labor case in the hospital and my order for pitocin augmentation was denied by a computer for a lack of some heart rate confirmation. I knew exactly what I was doing. I had been doing it pretty successfully for forty-three years! The computer was only two weeks in operation. But who can fight city hall or a machine hard drive? ♦

It didn't take long for the courts to get involved, including the Supreme Court. There have been several decisions passed down from on high that ensure that clients/patients cannot sue their HMOs for refusing to pay for doctor-recommended care. The far-reaching implications of such a ruling are too broad and vague to predict what will happen in the future.

These are some of the many decisions handed down by the Supreme Court that continue to keep the HMO and its parent insurance company essentially impervious from any accusations of wrongdoing and legal liability. The physician community is screaming at its highest decibel in protest. Especially as medical malpractice fees continue to go up and up and the physicians feel, legitimately, that they are taking the brunt of the rising costs of medical care on all levels.

It All Seemed to Happen So Suddenly

It seems as if it sure did take place overnight. The impact of the burgeoning HMO system came on like a veritable tsunami, and the doctor community got swept up in the roaring tide. Part of it was because the public was starving for a national healthcare plan and any change offered seemed an improvement. What struck us as the logic and wonders of Medicare and Medicaid were hoped for again.

There are all too many who know better who are working as activists and do-gooders in the movement to bring about healthcare for everyone. But they are as well quick to defend their precious Medicare and Medicaid, always footnoting any criticism of the status quo with a reminder that we should "...not knock Medicaid—it has been my life saver."

You only have to come back for a revisit to get their reaction when they are lopped off the Medicaid rolls or end up with shabby treatment such that they awaken to the grim facts that what we have, in whatever forms, just ain't enough.

Bob ran to the emergency room. He had done that a few times before. Every once in a while, his asthma catches him unawares and his inhaler pump just dries up. He was desperate. Worse, when he checked in at the front desk, the clerk—after a few punches into the computer—told him, rather glibly, that he was no longer registered and his Medicaid had lapsed. Then it hit him—he had taken a job in the past holiday season and made a little extra cash, finally. He did great. But that blew his Medicaid coverage.

This was on a Sunday afternoon, and he was not able to get in to see a Medicaid counselor until the following morning. He just panted until then. He got a temporary pass to get his pump, but now he's always afraid it will happen again. ♦

After executive "ambassador" Hillary Rodham Clinton met with the heads of the insurance industry, the doctors were told to take "two HMOs and call me in the morning." The HMOs then sold their bill of goods to corporate America, promising to save it millions in employee insurance premiums.

And the good old family docs, and then the specialists? They were transformed into cloying, sanctimonious antiques that spent too much time with patients, ordered too many ancillary tests, and made medical costs soar. Demonization again won out. Doctors and their patients again lost.

Those DRGs, gatekeepers, and carve outs, for starters, quickly replaced the outmoded practitioners. With the explosion of HMOs came rules and regulations, and when the smoke cleared, the physicians had surrendered their patient responsibilities to people practicing medicine without a license, holding an MBA instead of an MD degree.

What has actually happened to doctors now that they have been upstaged by the HMOs and their insurance company parents? Time was when our physicians were at the pinnacle of society. They were the guests of honor at town meetings and social events; they were either presidents of the local country club, the Kiwanis, or the Elks and were always recognized and honored from the podium at the high school graduation ceremonies.

With the vast majority of insurance-covered employees' (over two-thirds) being members of an HMO by 2006, and with that number climbing, HMO/managed care is slowly but surely becoming identified as the American standard and hallmark. The healthcare dollar has not fallen an iota; the proceeds have just shifted from the doctors/providers to their HMO partners/overseers.

The doctors'/providers' resentment can be cut with a scalpel. They ceded their patients to the HMOs before realizing what was happening and even agreed to pay for the shipping and handling.

CHAPTER 7

The Pharmaceuticals Need a Pill: The Plight of Prescription Drugs in America

Viagra is an obscene and shameful drug. Not because it was an entry into the pharmaceutical armamentarium that would help men and couples combating erectile dysfunction and often get them past a very difficult and sensitive moment in their lives. It is nice, indeed, that we now have something that will make love, not war. What is obscene and shameful is that Pfizer's costs to produce a ten milligram (mgm) Viagra pill, a standard dose, can be measured in pennies practically, but they sell it for at least ten dollars, usually more, at the drug counter.

And the more they sell the cheaper it is to produce. But the price at the counter stays put. Don't look for a competitive price. There are several choices for treatment out there now, but they are all cost the same. To the penny. They all shook hands on that one. Viagra (et al) is an obscene and shameful drug.

So how would you like to be in a business that has a twenty-times or even more markup as compared to just about every other manufacturer in the U.S.? GM, GE, IBM, and Panasonic, at their levels, are content to come in with a profit markup of about 1 to 3 percent on their autos, refrigerators, computers, and TV sets. Their volume makes them their billions. Sherman antitrust, where are you when we need you?

The pharmaceutical companies don't stop there. They charge many times that and more. They go unchecked as to what prices they set, despite the importance of their products. And all the pharmaceutical houses are members of the same club. Country club, that is.

Indeed, once a price is set with all the buyer can bear, the next company knows how much to put aside for promotion and packaging. When those so-called "competitors" are announced, the price being charged is for the medical concept and promise of treatment, rather than actual costs of production. There are no other variables. Again, Sherman antitrust—where are you?

Big Pharma and the R & D Myth

Many myths abound about the pharmaceutical industry. Where to start debunking them is the only question. It is an industry that seemingly has no saving grace or boundaries. There was a Gallup Poll several years ago that rated those professions and careers that were most trusted by the American people. Needless to say, used car salespeople, politicians, and lawyers shared the bottom of the list. Doctors were not at the top, but not at the bottom either—they were high midway in the list of twenty. Sadly, police officers were not as high up as I would hope. I guess reaction to that profession depended on social factors. If you were ever ticketed for DWB (driving while black), the beat cop lost a lot of points.

The corner pharmacist headed the list, and perhaps for good reason. Even by law, druggists, as they were once called, are more responsible than people realize. If the doctor writes a prescription that is more than illegible—it is of a dose or has an instruction that is improper or even dead wrong (no pun intended)—the pharmacist is obligated to refuse to fill it until he/she checks with the physician and confirms both dosing and indication. Many a time a decimal point for the dosage gets misplaced by the busy clinician or, if there had been some sort of emergency or urgency, there might have been confusion during the patient visit. It has happened to many a doctor. The pharmacist would be held responsible if any serious consequences had resulted. Doctors count on the promise that the pharmacist will stay alert.

Just about the biggest myth of all is the one most often put forward by drug house reps peddling in the doctors' offices or while pushing their PR plans: Yes, there may indeed be wider markup for their products as compared to other manufacturers, even a very wide markup. But that is all necessary, we are told, because of the enormous costs of so-called research and development (R & D) that goes into the preparation for the agent. Years and years of intricate and expensive lab research, animal testing, and human trials are needed before the U.S. Food and Drug Administration (FDA), the watchdog agency that is wholly responsible to the public at large for the safety and efficacy of a drug, will allow it to reach the marketplace.

But they don't tell us the rest of the story. Any number of studies have shown that at least 75 percent, and depending on the type of drug involved, up to as much as 90 percent, of the R & D costs are borne not by the drug houses but by the taxpayers in the form of National Institutes of Health (NIH) subsidization or specially issued Congressional grants to NIH or other governmental agency labs for exactly that—the R & D. The pharmaceutical lobbies a long time ago successfully worked the Hill for the federal government to bear the brunt of the R & D. Wait, it gets worse.

If the research, investigations, development, or animal and human trials do not result in a useful product from certain efforts, the program is simply abandoned, as it should be. We never hear about most of them. But, and here's the kicker, if all of that ends up in a useful and valuable agent, the rights and control of the materials, data, and the product totally revert to the drug company, including all patents.

Oh, yes, there is one more thing that goes to the drug company: all future profits from the sales. Only the promo and advertising campaigns are the private pharmaceuticals' responsibilities.

How would you like to be in a business that has the bulk of your overhead of costly R & D taken care of by the feds (read: taxpayers) and all you have to do is sit back, wait for one of them to work out, and move in to gather the profits that roll in? That is still happening to this very day, and despite this now having become well known, drug company spokespersons still ply their innuendos that R & D is at company expense.

Generic Myths

Yet another major facet of the drug business is the generics that came into vogue after World War II. Before then, their production had only been sporadic. As the country reverted to a peacetime mode in all industries, the pharmaceuticals turned their attention to consumer products. At first, the major players in the business scoffed at the impact the generics would make. They were convinced their reputation and relationship with America's medical community were safe.

And in part, that was true. Three-martini lunches, third-row-center theatre tickets for the doctor and spouse. Even an occasional weekend to some glamorous resort hotel with a golf tournament and tennis match mingled in with a lecture series and scientific session kept the docs more or less in line. But generics started to make more and more noise by the sixties.

In 1968, Richard Nixon was recovering from his earlier campaign waged for the California senate and his losses to John Kennedy for the presidency in 1960 and the governorship of California in 1962. It was going to be a close race for the White House, what with his past and the nationwide unrest over the ongoing Vietnam conflict, by then in full storm.

Nixon's inner circle included one Elmer Bobst, then-CEO at Warner-Lambert, later merged and known as Warner-Chilcott, a major player in the pharmaceutical industry. A vice-presidential running mate had to be carefully chosen, and preferably one removed politically from the Vietnam debate. Bobst had the solution.

The Maryland legislature was about to vote on allowing generics in the state to gain a new presence. It was feared, with good reason, that if and when this proved to be beneficial to the drug consumers, other states would quickly follow suit. Medicare was still embryonic, only three years old, and without any medications being covered, fixed-income seniors would get needed relief at the drug counters. There loomed a potential loss in revenue to the pharmaceuticals in the billions. Bobst, a long-time political conservative, a GOP faithful, and supporter of the Nixon camp, grabbed the reigns.

In a smoke-filled very private meeting with candidate Nixon and his inner circle, Bobst took out his Warner-Lambert's checkbook and made an offer that the Grand Old Party could not refuse. For enough zeros written after any given number on the check, he extracted the privilege of naming the VP candidate, assuring the GOP it would be someone untainted by an Indochina odor. A handshake followed and the fix was in. Bobst smiled broadly.

He then hopped into his limo for the hour-long ride to Annapolis and met with the then obscure Maryland Governor Spiro

Agnew. Bobst knew his pigeon well. Agnew had likely reached the pinnacle of his political career. His already established shady reputation got him a high state office, but a national spot was probably unattainable. Bobst made him that offer that was certainly not refused.

For a veto of the upcoming Maryland vote for the generics, and one that was veto-proof, Bobst dangled the vice-presidency. As the U.S. Communist Party political annals relate the story, Bobst wasted no time. An immediate call back to Washington assured all that the deal was set. Cash the check. The rest is history.

The Nixon-Agnew ticket eked by for the election victory and even won a second term by a wide margin in 1972, later on demeaned by the Agnew resignation under a dark cloud of cash kick-backs and the Watergate debacle that cost Nixon his place in the Oval Office and any credibility in U.S. history books.

But it had served its purpose well for Bobst and the pharmaceuticals. The Maryland defeat of the generic law stopped the hemorrhage; many other states waiting in the wings held back. It was several years later that the generics gained some legal credibility. The estimate of financial gain by Bobst, Warner-Lambert-Chilcott, and the others was well worth the hefty price tag for the GOP coffers. Its legacy included a slow down for the independent drug houses for many more years. It was money well spent. Regrets have never been mentioned. ♦

Enter the FDA

The generics, although gaining in popularity with the consumer and druggist, are still running into roadblocks along their way to you, and the structure of many states' statutes tries to halt their flow. The patent, no matter how derived, gives the brand name a seven-year holiday before a generic can be introduced. When it is finally time, the formulas of the newly discovered compounds, documented in FDA files, can be copied with certain restrictions and the clinical guarantees must be strictly met in order to call it a generic of a brand drug.

Brand spokespersons continually harp on this practice as a selling point for their wares—that even the slightest alteration in chemical formula potentially, or in reality, changes the drug's function, rendering it useless or even detrimental.

Doctors often remain wary until given absolute assurance and sometimes even wait a time for patient use and acceptance, and then, success of treatment. All prescription blanks now include a lower box in which the prescribing clinician must indicate if the brand is demanded or a generic is allowed. When not marked, the pharmacist will use the option of either, of course choosing the one with the greater markup.

Opening remarks during a recent pharmaceutical board meeting: Remember, our only mission is to extend lives. Of patients? No, of patents. ♦

But that formula manipulation that cannot be copied exactly is a subterfuge of another order. One trick, for example, used by the brandmakers, plays out frequently. Since there is that seven-year grace period before generics can be introduced into the marketplace, a particular drug put on the retail shelves stands alone. But the clock begins to tick, though too slowly for some. Impatient, a competitor house will examine the agent, take advantage of the years of study and bureaucracy by the company of origin, and play games with the formula. A simple and essentially meaningless switch of a single carbon atom or valence barrier, for example, will be sufficient to overcome the patent protection laws.

With a new name, packaging, and sales presentation, a my-drug-is-better-than-your-drug pitch is made to the doctor, and a new seven-year delay for generics starts a new timetable. These "me-too" drugs have become common in the industry. A new study that compares the newer concoction with the older, always purporting a marked improvement in results and side effects, is then announced with pride. Only the costs at the drug store counter remain the same and as high.

And we know that, from time to time, there comes about embarrassing exposures of a medical school/center investigative lab that took a hefty grant from the drug company or NIH to be less-than-genuine about the findings. Heads roll, the investigating researcher gets reprimanded, the public affairs department at the center gives out their most eloquent "No comment" to the press, and the band plays on. It is all part of the "publish or perish" practices of university medical empires. The most prestigious and wealthy institutions are not impervious. Maybe that is one way they got so wealthy.

The FDA has a long and circuitous history. Our founding fathers (and some mothers by then) sensed early on that some form of drug regulation was needed as the United States of America was unfolding. It was in 1820, when we were barely fifty years old, with a population of not quite 10 million and a geographical center in West Virginia, that the new nation established the U.S. Pharmacopoeia that set national drug standards. In 1862, President Abraham Lincoln created the Division of Chemistry at the Department of Agriculture, the direct forerunner to the FDA.

At the start of the twentieth century, Congress felt that "quack drugs" had to be controlled and a specific agency was to be assigned the task. In 1927, the Food and Drug Administration was officially born.

The Food, Drug, and Cosmetic Act was passed in 1938, regulating medical devices and cosmetics. Over-the-counter (OTC) drugs had to have appropriate labels for patient protection, and the FDA added dates and doses on so-called addictive meds to control so-called addicts. The U.S. Pharmacopoeia had made drastic changes in the laws in 1920, and such addictive street drugs as cocaine and heroin and their derivatives were deemed illegal across the board. Up to then, cocaine was a frequent additive to many cough preparations and assorted other household remedies.

In 1941, the FDA was moved under the aegis of the Federal Security Agency, but that was then abandoned in 1953 to become a cabinet post, the Department of Health, Education, and Welfare, where it has found a permanent home.

The machinery for a new drug varies, of course, but essentially follows a set of given rules. The drug house chemists will conceive an idea for an agent and its indications. Sometimes, they have been known to come up with an agent that makes chemical and clinical sense and then invent an indication for its use. The one most bantered about is for the drug methylphenidate (brand name: Ritalin). The agent was introduced and, admittedly, had no known indication or need. The concept of Attention Deficit Disorder (ADD) in children was then added to the formulary and voila! the drug found a home.

"Your condition has no symptoms or health risks, but there is a great new pill for it." ♦

The collaboration with NIH or other federal labs and medical arms is made and the chemistry is studied and honed for use. Then comes the animal testing, often almost silly in its application. Lower animal tests are a sine qua non of the FDA, even though some of that data is not transferable to humans.

For example, mood-altering and emotional-behavior agents cannot obviously be tested in lab specimens, whether they are rodents or mammals or whatever. Also suspect are those animals that have such different physiology that the information gained may be either useless or harmful. It is difficult to imagine that by giving a drug agent to, for example, a rodent that lives in a sewer and survives on eating vermin and sewage, a researcher can translate those side effects to the human model.

Some years ago, tragically, a repair method and drug were tested for narrow-angle glaucoma in rabbits. First, the condition was created in the rabbit by a surgical manipulation. When the management proved successful, the same manipulation and drug were used on several humans in a major and prestigious medical institution. The human subjects all went blind. It was later realized that the rabbit cornea's morphology and anatomy were different to the point that the tests were obviously aberrant. The data was not applicable to the homo sapiens. Lawsuits ensued, as expected. ♦

Nonetheless, animal tests continue in every FDA application in the hopes that some benefits can be gained when properly selective. That is followed by human trials, without which the agent cannot be introduced to the market place. The labs, the drug companies, and even the NIH must find enough human subjects to accept medications and procedures that have not been proven to be proper or indicated and accept the harsh potential risks that may accompany such unevaluated drugs. Where do they find takers? The answer is sadly obvious—the Third World, either domestic or foreign.

Insidious Racism

Just about all human drug investigations are carried out in public hospitals, Third World Latin America, or other Third World nations wherever. I leave it to your imagination if the subjects are made aware of what they are being given or what is about to happen to them. There is the imprimatur that is always added to such reports that the patients (read: subjects) had been given some financial rewards and an informed consent form in their native language for signing.

But study after study has revealed that maybe the money was offered, just maybe; the informed consent is another matter. With the literacy rate at alarmingly low levels that leaves as many as half of the subjects without the ability to read or write, and with the glamour of that paltry few dollars as a glaring temptation, it is no wonder these people would sign for anything against their best interests or health.

There are those other significant and now well-publicized studies and experiments that can only be described as cruel and vicious. At the turn of the twentieth century, almost 2,000 subjects with syphilis were withheld established treatment in Oslo, Norway, in order to follow the natural course of the disease.

Three decades later, the infamous Tuskegee prison study did the same to black prison inmates in Alabama. And just in case you think these are tied to the racism that is assumed to have been relegated to the history books, in 1990 to 2000, a series of New York City black and Hispanic school children with AIDS exposure and confirmed diagnoses were also denied known treatments, again to follow and study the pathology.

Racism and colonialism remain alive and well in the twenty-first century. Today, U.S. and other Western pharmaceutical companies test even the drugs that are considered relatively benign over-the-counter medications such as antacids, aspirins, and cold medicines in Third World countries, mainly in South America and Africa. Only those colonial nations such as India, with their own flourishing pharmaceutical manufacturing that is producing generics for use in the Western world, sometimes including the United States, use their own human patients as a testing ground for the products. But the U.S./FDA often rejects these pharmaceuticals as being unsafe and insecure for human usage.

This is frequently debated in Congress. On one side are those who suggest that India-produced medicines are being withheld because of their competition to the brands in the U.S.; the other side insists that the FDA and the Congresspeople are concerned about the validity and efficacy of these meds when they come from outside of U.S. plants and testing labs.

After the human trials are complete, the results are presented to FDA panels that then rule on whether the agent will be allowed into the U.S. marketplace. It should come as no surprise that the drug house lobbies are plentiful and powerful up on Capitol Hill. Frequently, when an approved and utilized medication eventually results in untoward and even serious side effects, even mortalities, exposed shabby and incomplete FDA testing were found to have accepted the drug for its approval. The most recent problems discovered with the class of drugs known as coxibs (Cox-2) are exemplary.

After years of wide use for relief from the pains and progression of rheumatoid and osteoarthritis, the Cox-2s on the market were found to cause deleterious cardiac side effects that had gone unmentioned in the drug warning portion of the package inserts and in the usual directives and pitches sent to physicians upon their introduction. One of the agents was removed from the market; the others were ordered to include updated curtailed prescriptions, and although being restudied and evaluated, the status of the medications remains in doubt.

But what surfaced from the uproar was that the Cox-2s were not screened or examined as closely as they might have been. The companies behind these medicines are heavyweights in the field. Data from less than 1,000 patients were used for the approval of Vioxx, the first Cox-2. Contrast that to what had taken place with the agent RU-486, the French oral abortifacient that went through years and years of intense evaluation and many thousands of patient subjects before it was released in 2000 by the FDA. There are strong indications that the fundamentalist right wings of both political parties were quite influential in the delay as a part of their campaign in the so-called anti-choice movement in the issue of abortion and choice.

A long-standing patient, Carol, called the office. Her voice was steady but I could hear the anxiety. She needed help. She told me she was several days pregnant and wanted my help in arranging for an abortion. I responded to her questions, asked a few of my own, and she seemed determined that RU-486 was the best approach. She mulled over the available options, but after conferring with her partner, decided to go the RU-486 route, against my advice. I instructed her to have her pharmacist call me for the prescription. She called me from the street a few hours later and told me her frustrating news. After no fewer than seven tries, no pharmacy had it in stock or readily available. This legal FDA-approved medication just could not be bought in New York City. Carol threw in the towel, and we collectively took care of the matter. ♦

The FDA has shown itself many times over to be quite inconsistent in its deliberations and decisions, and the distinct influence exerted by the drug industry has always been evident. However, there certainly have been rewarding moments in FDA history that have buoyed it up. Caution an era ago prevented the import of the German drug thalidomide, which caused serious birth defects in Western Europe. It was never used in the U.S., with great credit to FDA alertness.

Back in the 1980s during a European working vacation, I made arrangements to meet up with a medical school classmate who had gone on to a specialty in pharmacology. His career eventually took him to a very successful pharmaceutical firm, Hoffman LaRoche. He moved up the corporate ladder to a vice-presidency. I renewed our close friendship with fond memories over dinner and cocktails and I, of course, accepted his invitation for a full service panorama of company headquarters. I just knew a real treat was in store.

We went through the labs, the production departments, shipping platforms, and even the administrative offices. It was as rewarding as expected. Near the end of the day's tour, my colleague turned to me and said, "Now we will visit the real power behind our success." I was confused. I thought I had seen it all but was about to learn otherwise.

The elevator door slid open to a "Sixth Floor" expanse filled with bright retractable lights, drawing tables, easels and artists' paraphernalia, camera and video equipment, and the like. There, hundreds of personnel were scattered about at their slanted tables with colored pencils and artists' brushes putting together ideas and schematics for the cartons and packaging for the products invented and polished on the floors above and below.

"Without the right name, box color, and logo, no matter how helpful the drug may be, it won't sell a lick. It must look right. This is where it all happens." My friend shared an anecdote from the history of his company that fortified his comments.

During the early stages of World War II, German scientists in the 1930s had put together the first breakthrough in what eventually came to be known as antibiotics, the next big discovery being the post-war introduction of penicillin. The rest is legendary history.

The agent was a yellow powder that was called sulfa, and one of its isomers, sulfanilamide, was immediately shipped off in large quantities to the battlefields as a wound antiseptic. Its success was marked and immediate. Allied chemists rushed in a frenzy to put their own analogue into service.

The FDA deserves a pat on the back for an action it took at this moment in its history. An elixir of sulfanilamide was found to have been contaminated with a toxin, and over 100 patients were fatally affected. The FDA reacted quickly and promptly halted its U.S. import.

The peacetime world awaited the application of sulfa. It was labeled "Sulfin," put into a blue box with the LaRoche logo, and peddled to doctors throughout the world as a urinary disinfectant. Its success was less than moderate.

LaRoche wondered what went wrong; the pharmacological value of the chemical was unmistakable. Then the "Sixth Floor" went into action. The name was changed to "Gantrisin" (no one at LaRoche seemed to know where that name had come from), the box color went from blue to yellow (the color of urine), and the company emblem was drawn less prominently. Within the next few years, it rose to become one of the world's best-selling medications. With good clinical reason. It worked.

Same drug, same indications, different packaging and name. Go figure.

Big Pharma Is Special in So Many Ways

Obviously, the pharmaceutical industry figures integrally into the dire straits of healthcare in America. It certainly fits into the Byzantine world of healthcare's social and political barriers.

For openers, the product itself cannot be considered extraneous. It has been said that we need it all, from a picture hook to an automobile tire patch, all of which have their purpose. When you want to hang a picture of Aunt Mary before her visit, that little hook and pin nail gimmick becomes priceless; and try finding a fix for a nail in the tire tread when you are on your way to Aunt Mary's for dinner.

But drugs stand alone. They are directly related to our lives and have no equal as a commercial product. For that reason, the profit margins and other forms of arrogance displayed by the drug industry have been so tolerated by the American public. And the eventual sales price, whether or not it is from a company that went to more expense for its development or one that changes a single hydroxyl molecule on carbon ring number fourteen and makes a "me-too" drug, stays the same. No one even challenges that rationale. The unsuspecting buying public is victim to a price fixing that is ubiquitous to the industry.

Take one of America's best-selling drugs, the female birth control pill (BCP)—that ingenious combination of the female hormones estrogen and progesterone that has serviced untold millions of women worldwide since 1960, one of the major progressive steps for women's health and control of their conception mechanism in the history of medicine. In one fell swoop, it put fertility into the decision-making hands of women, the gender that bears the physical and social brunt of a pregnancy and the offspring, planned or otherwise.

Upon its development in the 1950s and introduction to the market ten years later, the dose was set at ten milligrams, soon reduced to five on the progesterone side. The estrogen moiety also went through a series of reductions as researchers discovered that the contraceptive effects of the "pill" could be achieved at a much lower dose.

Yet, despite the competition from those same hormones being delivered by other means, such as injection, dermal patches, and vaginal rings, the oral contraceptive agent (OCA/BCP) stays near the top of the charts in sales. The hormones themselves have actually not basically changed, altered with only minor molecular variations in the original chemical formula.

Yet, even though the pharmaceutical production lines can often derive as many as hundreds more doses from that ten mgm amount of 1960, the cost to the consumer has not changed a penny. In fact, there have been increases over and above inflation indices that are always attributed to that mythical "research and development." "Me-too" OCPs are introduced regularly, always with the claim for a new sensational breakthrough that makes it better than last year's. The new patent on what is then sold to women as a new product earns it another seven years' protection before generics can get into the act. There is no end in sight.

Overheard said by the pharmacist at the drug counter. "The drug itself has no serious, bad side effects, but the price may cause dizziness and fainting spells." ♦

The influence held over the FDA by the mammoth and even smaller pharmaceuticals is the stuff of legends. In Washington, their lobbies are considered among the strongest and most vociferous, right up there with the Israeli and gun lobbies. All three are quite successful. Just look it up.

Allegedly, the FDA has built-in watchdogs. There are various committees within that are charged with second looks after a drug has been approved and may even have been on the retail shelves for some time. These committees have the power to review and even cancel approval when deemed necessary. That happens every once in a while, though certainly not often enough.

Many agents, like the Cox-2s, got by the original unit in the FDA for release approval. The trouble remains that the approval committee and the watchdog unit are under the same leadership, command, and payroll. Many an FDA whistle-blower has admitted that you don't "poop where you eat."

Recent reports have shown that almost 50 percent of the agency's nearly half-billion-dollar budget is paid for by the drug industry. This took a big jump in the early 1990s when research for AIDS reached its height; supposedly, the funds were intended to speed the process for HIV treatments. The "user fees" provided to the drug companies to administer their untried formulations on Third World "guinea pigs" have not dried up. Spokespersons from the Pharmaceutical Research and Manufacturers of America (Pharma), the industry's trade-group, report this with a certain pride.

The marriage between the FDA and the drug houses and even a group of prestigious medical journals is clear and obvious, not just rumored. A former editor of the *NEJM*, certainly among the nation's most respected publications, stated "[that there were] large-scale breaching of the boundaries between academic and for profit industry." Dr. Marcia Angell, author of a current exposé of the drug companies' questionable trading practices, called for renewed efforts to disallow academic researchers from investing in companies whose drugs they research. Financial support by the pharmaceutical industry of medical schools and their journals is common knowledge.

A recent study as reported in *The Observer* out of the UK, inquired into the validity of the many articles appearing in renowned British medical journals claiming to be written by academics or investigating physicians on medical school faculties and at research centers. Publications by medical literati are international in scope and acceptance. The findings were more than alarming. The study revealed that many of the alleged studies and research projects were actually penned by paid-for-hire ghostwriters with an assignment to plug the product being evaluated. You can just imagine what happened to the data that would prove to be in any way unfavorable.

The doctors and other highly degreed researchers were then plugged in as authors. *The Observer* study showed there were several articles published under the byline of a physician or doctor of the medical sciences who was actually employed by the drug company, and was anything but an independent observer.

Doctor Richard Smith, editor of the *British Journal of Medicine*, admitted that ghostwriting was a "...very big problem. We are often being hoodwinked by the companies. Hopefully we find out in time and reject the paper. When we...[insist] any involvement by a drug company should be made explicit...they found ways...to go undercover."

Reaching Out to Consumers: DTC Advertising

Another sign of the complacency the drug industry expects and enjoys in Washington, safe in the knowledge that their three-martini lunches are paying off up in the Senate Office Building and the Oval Office, is the recent advent of direct-to-consumer (DTC) advertising. TV and lay journal advertising are in. This rapidly became a $3 billion marketing industry, and climbing. It seems to take a setback every once in a while when the FDA does catch-up with an illicit product, like the Cox-2s, for example. But there is always a speedy recovery. New markets are constantly being tapped.

DTC is unquestionably successful—if you measure success by sales. You will be seeing more and more of it in the near future. The drug company obviously claims that the ads are educational to a buying public; the other guys say that such marketing can easily result in an exertion of pressure upon physicians to prescribe medicines otherwise not used, and it may even increase sales of riskier and more expensive products. The success of the Cox-2 Vioxx, now discredited and off the market, came after a whirlwind blitz of super-duper TV, magazine, and newspaper ads.

The implications are clear. When sports icons, Hollywood and matinee idols, and even high-up elected officials recommend something, the subliminal message is there for all to see. If those important people, with their wherewithal to get what they want, take this or that, it must be the best. It works with jeans, cosmetics, soda pop, and breakfast cereal, so why not medications? No reason.

DTC ads are misleading in many ways. Yes, they do spend some airtime describing various untoward side effects and even contraindications, always making sure they are seemingly unpleasantries, expectant and casual. In the old days, however, a reputable medical journal article would codify and a legitimate investigating clinician would discuss medications with a patient, their pros and cons, and pick the best one for the treatable pathology. TV ads obviously will not give you two sides. They are sales pitches, pure and simple. That TV time costs real bucks.

Certainly, by creating a patient demand, the ads ensure that doctors will feel the squeeze to prescribe as the path of least resistance. This saves lots of time per visit and, when the physician is getting reimbursed by some HMO capitation or set fee, a bad habit is being formed in the office. There is also the problem that when patients start lecturing the doctor on what was heard during the breaks in a favorite TV sitcom, it can be embarrassing for the doctor-authority not to know it all, so, accepting the come-on, a written prescription is offered. It becomes a "shared decision," when it was actually made by the TV pitch and the buying patient. The doctor is truly a mere provider.

Take the GI relief agent Prilosec, by AstraZeneca. It was at one time the leading medication in sales in the U.S.. As the generics were moving in, AstraZeneca started promoting "me-too" Nexium, an almost identical drug, with one or two of those carbon atoms changed in its formula. Oh yeah, AstraZeneca's "Sixth Floor" went to work and changed the logo and packaging color. The advent of a whole lot of less expensive generic Prilosecs was about to cut into AstraZeneca's profits by the many millions. Nexium averted the problem. Other examples by the other houses abound. ♦

Such DTC promotions follow the ethics of the advertising world, manipulating people into buying things they really don't need or even want. It is all part of the gestalt of HMO medicine. MBAs instead of MDs are ordering tests and management and making diagnoses; TV hucksters are manipulating consumer brain waves into making decisions as to what is the best agent for whatever ails them. The sobriquet that calls the doctor a provider is apt.

Pretty soon, the obvious will be part of the company mystique. Just as the industry uses that mythical R & D clamor to justify the markup, the truth be damned, now will be added a plea to cover the costs of those consumer ads, and the ads will be justified to build sales to increase a need to augment a factory output that will give them the volume to reduce prices.

Demand? Yes. Sales? Yes. Volume? Yes. Profits? For sure. Price reduction? Uh-huh. Don't hold your breath. Ain't happened yet.

The Drug Lobby

There is no better example of why healthcare must be taken out of the for-profit private sector than to paint the bottom line on prescription drugs. More than one study, from the Public Citizen (PC) onward, has revealed that those much more expensive drugs launched by a costly TV ad series with expensive glamour girls and noted celebrities do not stack up clinically when tested against other meds that do the same job for a fraction of the cost and do not need any DTC campaigns.

I remind you that this is not some new automobile, laundry detergent, or hair shampoo we are talking about but a life-saving medication. A little different, don't you think? Just some food for thought.

Investigative reporter Marc Siegel, with tongue-in-cheek, put it this way. During the last Super Bowl with those ads going for a million dollars and more per minute, he told of a viewer who was so impressed with the glamorous pitch-people selling an OTC "antidepressant" type of drug that he went out and bought some, even though he wasn't feeling depressed. Then, when he developed an erectile dysfunction side effect, he had to buy into the ads for the ED relief. "That is how the system works," Siegel sadly concluded. "That's how it works on people." ♦

Another cog in the machine of DTC hawking is the blooming and booming pills-by-mail or pills-over-the-Internet. Some savings are being passed on to the consumer, as the overhead of the electronics is less than having to open a storefront in a high-rent urban center or mall and hiring humans, including pharmacists, to patrol the counters. As you might expect, the humongous drug chains are able to compete and are even a part of that empire.

The mom and pop drug stores, also as expected, are getting it stuck to them in yet another way. They can't compete with the chains and certainly not with the order-by-mail people. Human beings in the doctors' offices and hospitals are being replaced by computers, monitor machines, and HMO officers many miles away; now the meds are being dispensed not by your friendly pharmacist but by an electronic mail-order or Internet robot.

There are other subtle downsides. The *Wall Street Journal* reported that the drug companies are certainly keeping their collective eyes on their bottom lines. If they can achieve what they want for their stockholders by selling more of what they have through DTC campaigns—or better, change that one chemical valence in the formula and make another "me-too" drug—there comes less of a need to get to their collective labs and find new and improved medications. The bottom line is the financial bottom line. The attitude is that how they get there is no one's business but theirs.

Stem cell research, tied in, of course, with the issue of abortion and choice, will take center stage in the news for the foreseeable future. The Bush Administration, under heavy fundamentalist influence, is on the con side. Guess who is there along with them. The pharmaceutical industry.

Having the ability in the future to run down to your replacement emporium for a new organ part that had been created from a stem-cell anlage may be a futuristic twenty-fifth-century Buck Rogers fantasy right now, but it's obviously an eventual reality. The concern by Big Pharma is that with fewer pathologic organs, fewer medicines will be needed for treatment.

But such a machinery will require a whole new host of agents needed to deal with the new organ immune responses. Reaching that conclusion unfortunately requires foresight not demonstrated by the pharmaceutical companies. With a bottom line and end-of-the-year statement to face, the time is now. The future will have to take care of itself.

The news is not all bad. There are glimmers of hope and relief for the consumers in individual states, but without a federal agenda, uniformity is hard to come by. Here we live in a nearly contiguous nation of fifty states, but yet, with some of these draconian drug laws and healthcare packages, it almost seems like you are in a foreign land when you cross a state line. Part of that is because the bulk of funds for the sad excuses for healthcare and medications that are state administered are funded by federal match, and (as with Medicaid and Medicare) each state house closely guards its coffers.

One of the exceptions that has a long history is what happened in New York after the turn of the twentieth century when immigration was reaching its pinnacle. As the Ellis Island gateway was opened and the USA was becoming the USA with its massive influx of immigrants, the state of New York and the federal immigration agencies realized that some of its state health regulations could not be translated to New York City because of its unusual size, growth, and scope. So a separate city department of health was created and, as long as it did not counteract state statutes, was permitted to revise and alter general health rules to fit those special needs. Some of the other states have followed in kind.

The International Prescription Drug Trade

Then there is the pressure exerted by consumers and pharmacies alike to seek out better deals on medications from abroad, notably Canada and Mexico, as well as any and everywhere else in the world. This became dramatized when the George W. Bush Administration started their Medicare revisions that further convoluted the way seniors were to get affordable drugs, with those mile-wide loopholes that protected the private pharmaceuticals, and even more Machiavellian restrictions on access.

Thus, drug imports from India, with its vast pharmaceutical plants, and Canada, known for its availability of less costly products, were barred. With India, it was easy to sell the public that the polluted conditions there would make the alien meds possibly contaminated. That was enough to scare off a lot of people.

The public was told, as a part of the demonization of the Canadian National Health Service, that Canadians from those areas across our northern border with geographic access to our major urban centers like Detroit and Seattle and Buffalo were flocking to get U.S. healthcare rather than trust their own. Anyone who believed that could be sold a piece of oceanfront property in downtown Kansas City. Kept a secret was the reverse flow of statesiders who crossed northward to get their prescription drugs from Canadian pharmacies.

Item: Consolidated Auto Company is moving its assembly plant from Detroit to Ottawa to take the benefits of the Canadian NHS that considerably reduces manufacturing costs of each car.

Item: International Rubber Company took advantage of that draconian NAFTA to open a tire plant in Mexico to use non-unionized Mexican workers.

Item: WorldWide Investment Company incorporates in the Cayman Islands to use its special corporate tax breaks.

Item: Maude Johnson from Detroit is questioned for crossing the border to Canada to buy her medications and is accused of being anti-American. ♦

Does it really sometimes take a billion dollars to come up with a new therapeutic agent? The very mainstream journal *Scientific American* asked that question. Its conclusion was noteworthy.

There was a good deal of evidence that brought on hardcore accusations that Big Pharma is inflating those R & D figures in order to first get a bigger kick in from the feds at NIH and Congress and then to justify its price scale. Part of that kick in from Washington is either in direct payouts or simply very adequate tax benefits that amount to the same thing. The bigger the numbers, the bigger the write-offs.

The drug people insist that less than a quarter of the sought after agents ever make it to the marketplace, and so all of their perks are needed to cover the failures. That myth of who pays for what always needs feeding.

And just about everybody from *Scientific American* on down reminds us that the data from the drug house never seems to jibe with the eventual accounting when the federal figures are released. Sometimes, the differences between company and government actuaries are embarrassingly wide. A drug company recently reported an expenditure of $897 million; the federal number came in at $122 million! I would say that is some very creative accounting.

Doctor Angell, in her review of the industry, listed many, many other contradictions. Her message was loud and clear. There are just about no boundaries that the drug companies adhere to or recognize.

Alan Sager, a professor at Boston University's School of Public Health, has made several studies of the drug industry. "It's a terror tactic. If you touch our profits, the laboratories will close and you'll all die," he said. He was accurately paraphrasing Big Pharma's callous message to the buying public.

Public Citizen reminds us that, though you keep hearing that just about any and all big firms that make up the Fortune 500 have their peaks and troughs, some even have a losing year or two, you also hear drug company profit and loss columns never seem to need red ink. And when it gets perilously close, meaning not having as big a profit year as anticipated, they simply nudge the price per pill up a little and tell the public how much more is needed for that mythical R & D. Like Sager said: touch our profits, and you will all die.

Maine and West Virginia have made louder noises than the others in this struggle. Maine's act was to put a maximum on all prescription drugs and keep them within the guidelines as set by the U.S. Department of Veterans Affairs. West Virginia's representatives at a 2005 conference on drug reform in Minnesota were the most outspoken and announced plans to create a machinery back home to deal with the problems of those rising costs.

And now, newly elected New Jersey Governor John Corzine has proposed a plan to vastly increase healthcare coverage for the uninsured in his state. There are many skeptics who have dismissed his plans outright, suggesting it appears like more Titanic deck chair shifting. But this may be a big loss for the nation as a whole. With the governor being somewhat healthcare conscious, his influence might have been put to the better national good in the Capitol than in a single state house in Trenton.

Similar rumbles are now being heard in South Carolina and Pennsylvania and elsewhere where state legislatures are as befuddled over their respective states' plights as they are seeing the manipulations in funds from Washington.

In a knee-jerk reflex, George W. Bush's then-Health and Human Services (HHS) Secretary Tommy Thomson went along with drug giant Bayer in 2001 regarding a multi-million pill order for its powerhouse antibiotic, Cipro. They all agreed on the terms of the sale. But it soon became known that generics, a year before the patent on Cipro would run out, could produce the needed medications in half the time and for half the cost. Bayer and Thomson were just too embarrassed not to yield. Bayer supplied the drug at a reduced, albeit very profitable, figure.

Monica just got to the airport in time to make her international flight to Rome from New York and was properly labeled a "runner," doing double time down that entry hallway to squeeze in just before the pilot ordered the door shut. But when she landed, she realized her haste had prevented her from grabbing her thyroid pills out of her checked-in bag to put into her purse. When the airline desk at Fiumicino informed Monica her luggage didn't make it in the rush, she had to wait at least a couple of days before it could be sent to her hotel on the Italian Riviera by messenger transport.

Her host came to the rescue. He extracted a favor from a doctor friend to write a cover prescription to keep Monica on keel. She went off to the local chimico, put the week's supply of meds in her purse, and waited for the tab.

When the euros, even with a poor exchange rate, came to less than what she paid for just a couple of pills at home, she made sure she was being charged for the week's worth. She seriously wondered if it were not cost effective to take occasional trips to the Riviera just to pick up a decent supply of her Rx needs. Monica toyed with the idea of approaching a travel agency to cook up a package deal that offers an all-inclusive tour of Florence and a Venice gondola ride, all paid for by the savings on tourist pharmacy shopping.

I bet that might just work. ♦

Tax Relief for the Pharmaceuticals

Along with profits, the prescription-drug industry is also setting records for lobbying activities and political campaign contributions, according to several reviews of the industry. A report by the reputable watchdog group PC stated that the drug business spends over $85 million annually on Congressional lobbies, up about 10 million per year since 1997, the same year the FDA began requiring TV ads include a mention of side effects.

The PC report noted that the drug industry has almost 300 lobbyists on its payroll, about one for every two members of Congress. It has increased its kick in to the political parties by over 50 percent each year, and 150 percent in a presidential election year. Both major parties get their share; the drug houses are taking no chances, and, like their counterparts elsewhere among the Fortune 500, play both sides of the fence, as though there were actually two sides. The spread is about three to one in favor of the GOP. Now that up in Congress it has been decided to add prescription drug coverage to Medicare, despite its apparent disingenuousness as revealed with the shenanigans swelling up around Medicare Part D, the vying for position by the various pharmaceutical house lobbies is creating a traffic jam.

The breaks offered Big Pharma go further. Tax breaks, that is. As a part of the America Jobs Creation Act signed into law by President George W. Bush in October 2004, drug firms were allowed a one-year window to return foreign profits to the United States at a 5.25 percent tax rate, compared with the standard 35 percent. Not exclusive only to drug makers, of course. But they have been the biggest beneficiaries because they seem to move profits overseas with relative ease.

The legal loopholes in the tax laws have always been used aggressively by the pharmacy guys. They report to the IRS that an inflated portion of product sales come from overseas markets, when in fact, they are truly U.S. American; raw products perhaps are put together in a Honduran Quonset hut, but ultimately the finished medicine is made on American soil. The amounts returned so far for the new rate are measured in the tens of billions of dollars. Nice piece of change no matter how you measure it.

The drug industry spends a higher percentage of its revenue on campaign contributions and lobbying in Washington than does any other enterprise. It just seems that everything the industry does has a price tag.

Trusting Big Pharma

Again, because the pharmaceuticals follow the ethics and morals of the rest of Big Business, their deviant activities seem to be exaggerated, if only because of their product and its vital need. When you buy a lemon of a car, you trade it in or get your money back; when you get a lemon of a medication or none at all, your life is at stake by definition. A refund cannot get back your health or your life.

No question about it. The pharmaceutical industry is a growth industry and there are signs that those pharmacists who are now enjoying that number-one ranking in the people's trust may be selling out their birthrights. There are signs the dike is starting to leak and it may take more than a little boy's finger to plug it up. Just as the pharmacist still ranks at or near the top in people's trust, better than half of a recent nationwide polled group did in no way share that trust with online. I guess that loss of human touch still resonates. Hands-on medicine and face-to-face pharmacy still certainly mean a lot to many.

As the companies strive for more and more and are getting heavier and heavier into consumer advertising, they are enlisting the aid of their local pharmacists. Collaborating with may be more like it.

The Pharmacy Rights Clearing House (PRCH), a consumer advocacy group, filed a lawsuit in September 2004 against a California supermarket giant for allegedly selling the private prescription drug information of its customers to the pharmaceutical companies. PRCH named several pharmacy heavyweights as co-defendants, including AstraZeneca, Eli Lilly, and GlaxoSmithKline, claiming the companies used the information to then promote their drugs through unsolicited calls and letters. California's privacy regulation laws were violated, for openers.

Big Pharma's PR is at its height these days. Actors in their ads sport long white coats, the symbol of purity. The implication is that those friendly faces will be seen at the corner drugstore, the place where the public still attached some form of integrity that remembered when there was a soda fountain and a lunch counter. There is a rude awakening. The bright lights of Big Business have replaced all this. Your medication is in aisle 6, next to the school supplies and laundry detergent. You're on your own.

Doctor Martha Crouch, a former biology professor at the University of Indiana, resigned from her role in a major project after she found out that biotechnology companies were co-opting her well-respected research for pure profit. ♦

Trust is starting to erode on all levels as the deck chairs go through more shifting while the ship is sinking. I doubt there is anyone out there in either the media, the government, or from among consumers who can actually explain what the Bush Administration has up its sleeve for Medicare drug regs, Part D, for instance. And what happens there and how it plays out will no doubt inspire them to arrange for the same manipulations with Medicaid. The HMOs will surely follow the leader.

A *Washington Post* report in April 2005 tried to explain away whether those beneficiaries with chronic disease needs will save money or not. Even arch conservative Senator Zell Miller (D-GA), whose voting record from the floor is strictly along GOP lines, felt a need to express concerns for the plight of the elderly when they wrestle with the Medicare drug benefits changes. It is that old adage come true—liars figure and figures lie.

Last year, at a fashionable Washington hotel ballroom, the spring charity circuit opened with a glittering black-tie event that featured congressmen's wives as guests. One of the keynoters was CEO Robert Essner from Wyeth Pharmaceuticals, a major player in the menopause relief drug business. Its flagship agent, Premarin, has been under attack for several years by the animal rights groups. With good reason.

The drug is produced from pregnant mares' urine (hence the name) whose extraction subjects the herd to abusive behavior in order to maximize its urine collection. It has been demonstrated that a synthetic substitute would be a clone in chemistry and function. Wyeth is still holding on to its natural product for one reason—as long as it is more economical to get it that way. The bottom line again.

Anyway, Essner presented the sponsoring group with a quarter-million-dollar donation check as a part of his soft sell for Wyeth and Premarin. There were grumbles from the crowd that expressed resentment over commercializing the evening gala. One skeptic, however, then reminded the ladies that their irritation might last only until they tell their husbands, who then would recount last year's Wyeth campaign contributions.

Down the Road

So where are we going with all this? The question is simple to pose. The answer is not that easy. How can we get the power-laden pharmaceutical empire to provide the American people with their products that are so vital for our lives and welfare at an affordable price and still be profitable enough? It is likely not doable, as an isolated change. That toe bone and head bone are still connected. Without a proper universal healthcare package, it is merely pure fantasy.

But, on the other hand, while we are waiting around for Washington to respond to our needs, can we afford not to attack that one segment of the problem? Besides, drugs are the fastest-growing sector of the healthcare business.

In clinic services, wherein just about all patients are either on Medicaid or Medicare (90 percent), those who are forced to answer the puzzlement at their ailments' lack of response to prescribed medications sheepishly admit that it is only because the Rx was never filled. If on Medicaid, there was no coverage when the agent was nonformulary, and the costs were beyond the patients' means. If on Medicare, it would be that the prescription was eliminated from the federal allowances or never was covered. Or that the confusion over Part D caused such frustration the patients just gave up and went without. And, as many of the Medicaid programs are going HMO, a drug allowed under the federal Medicaid may not be so under the HMO Medicaid. The clinician never gets to know that until the patient comes back for that next visit. Too late.

Greed is the distinguishing feature of the international drug cartels. The disinformation is enormous, whether it is about "faulty" Indian and Canadian drugs, or the direct intimidation of a vulnerable population. And when you are poor and dependent on the public dole, you are vulnerable. Those hefty campaign contributions are more than enough to keep control over the governmental machinery, so the impoverished have learned not to turn to their representatives for any help.

Privatization is high on the Bush and future GOP agenda—in education, already underway; Social Security, in for the big push; and healthcare, well in tow. The drug coverages will be the tail behind the dog's wagging head. Medicare's Part D has that distinct privatization imprimatur with federal funds going to the pharmaceuticals that then dispense the prescription drugs to the enrollee.

It is being labeled medical marketing. The Wyeth dinner gala is one of many enticements. Money like that is being strewn around, buying influence and the status quo. Three-martini lunches or buying off a governor to make him a vice-president; they are just different ends of the same pole.

Prescription prices are really way up there.

Yes, but that is because of those costs for R & D.

R & D? What's R & D?

Rapacity and dishonesty. ♦

It has been estimated, at a low figure, that more than 20,000 Americans die yearly only because of a lack of needed medications to treat their illnesses. Yes, that is dwarfed by the nearly 10,000 who die every single day in the undeveloped countries of the world of AIDS only because treatments are just too expensive, or the hundreds of thousands who succumb to malaria for the lack of pennies worth of a curing dose of quinine. But three wrongs don't make a right.

The respected Seattle-based actuarial firm Milliman Medical Index (MMI) states that a 2005 family of four's average medical costs in the USA are over $1,000 a month. That was an almost 10 percent increase from 2004. The MMI spokesperson added that this is a burden that will be handled by less and less of the American public. MMI was taking into consideration what Washington has in store for our futures. And medications are the largest single portion of that load.

The pharmaceutical industry as we now know it has its own prescription for profit. It is as good as any a place to start for reform as we mobilize our forces to achieve full and universal healthcare for all. We will have to give it two pills and have it call us in the morning.

CHAPTER 8

The Business of Healthcare is Business: Doctors & Patients vs. HMOs & Hospitals

It was President Dwight D. Eisenhower's secretary of defense, conscripted CEO at General Motors aptly called "GM" Charlie Wilson, who said in 1952, "What's good for General Motors is good for America." Well, he may not have actually said it so succinctly, but he sure believed it and practiced it. Perhaps he was just taking a page out of the 1925 speech by then-President Calvin "Silent Cal" Coolidge who did say, "The business of America is business."

The start of the twenty-first century witnessed the biggest push in our history toward that fix. And that meant that every last tenet of public services was in big capital's line of fire. "Privatization" became the catchword. President George W. Bush, in more than one oration, described his goal for the country—making us a "nation of owners." But that is like saying the kid who runs a lemonade stand on the front lawn is a business mogul.

The march toward privatization is still on. It started back at the beginning of President Franklin D. Roosevelt's first term in the early 1930s, as we were trying to shake the abyss we came to know as the Great Depression, when privatization had reached its height. FDR was somewhat embarrassed when the Supreme Court struck down more than one of his New Deal programs that put the country back to work. But he "laughed all the way to the bank." He had already accomplished what he had set out to do—save the USA.

Perhaps his greatest coup was to hand out a little embarrassment of his own to the capital world of private enterprise after it refused to take on a project that would harness the rivers in the South in order to bring to those states much needed affordable electric power—and the jobs that went with it. His brilliant Secretary of Labor, Frances Perkins, again stepped into the fray as she had done so often in the past, and the two of them drew up the blueprints for the Tennessee Valley Authority which showed that a government with the right priority can do what private entrepreneurs could and would not. It did take giving up the huge profits that had been demanded by the private electrical contractors who were unwilling to work for less. To this very day, the TVA is pumping out the power and light that brought the South into the twenty-first century.

Electricity, telephones, natural gas, and even public transportation were put into a special category. This was Washington's way of compromising with Big Business—pointing out that certain services, like electric power and communications, were just too vital for our daily lives and, during a national emergency or disaster, could not be in the hands of the privateers.

Yes, there would be stockholders with their places on the stock exchanges of Wall Street, and there would be a bottom line. After all, there was that high judiciary still looming in the wings waiting to protect free enterprise from Karl Marx's specter that was haunting Europe. Remember? And "Silent Cal's" words were as true as ever. But the nature of those industries demanded and needed closer scrutiny. Ergo, the public utility concept was devised and put into operation.

We are now all seeing the next page in that book of aspirations. Public education, already privatized in many communities with predictable no-better-off results, is in for the big haul. And the next several years will likely be taken up by debates during election campaigns and on the floors of both houses of Congress deciding the fate of what is not so arguable as our most precious social accomplishment and holdover from FDR's New Deal—Social Security. The jury is still way out on that one.

Healthcare was always eyed with great lust. Hospitals were one of the last bastions to hold out against the onslaught of corporate America. The impetus toward national healthcare got underway in the first half of the twentieth century with failed attempts that were tied into Social Security and then took off an era later with the onset of managed care and the HMOs. The insurance industry licked its proverbial chops over the prospect of gobbling up the largest piece of the healthcare pie along with the pharmaceuticals—America's hospitals. This was the second coming of the gold rush.

The Classification of U.S. Hospitals

There are about 6,500 hospitals and about 16,000 nursing homes in America. That translates to almost one million hospital beds in the nation. By far, the majority of the hospitals are "general" hospitals in which a comprehensive range of ailments is treated.

About 1,000 hospitals fall into the category of "specialized" treatment centers, labeled as the pathology itself, like cardiac, renal, gynecologic and obstetric, cancer, etc. Super-specialized hospital centers can be dedicated as pulmonary sanitariums; cardiac units; burn centers; lying-in infirmaries; orthopedics-only, gynecology-only, oncology-only and radiology-only clinics, or to patient demographics—children, the elderly, or halfway rehab. Many a medical staff conference starts out with some wry humor that describes left and right lung and kidney treatment units and maybe left and right eye lazarettos, to carry this from the sublime to the ridiculous. In reality, the highly specialized hospitals have the facilities and equipment to meet their clinical needs and the trained staff to handle the most intricate and intense situations.

Most of the health-buying public is coming to realize that hospitals are different from one another on many levels, from size and facilities to personnel and temperament. According to the American Hospital Association (AHA), there are two major criteria that give hospitals their status—how narrowly specialized is their care and whether it is a formal teaching hospital. The teaching hospitals are usually associated and integrated with an adjoining medical school and have the attending staff members' holding didactic or clinical faculty positions. Those medical school affiliates are usually much larger and are tuned in to being teaching sites for all ranges of healthcare professionals, from practical nurses and lab technicians to registered nurses and physicians. Their sophistication can be a drawback or benefit, depending on a myriad of other issues and needs. Non-teaching hospitals, also known as community hospitals, have the advantage of being less costly and often less bureaucratically demanding.

A third category for rating has been added by various consumer groups, especially in this era of commercialism: whether the hospital is nonprofit or for-profit. That depends on one question—who owns the hospital? They fall into three categories.

A voluntary hospital is essentially a not-for-profit community facility operating under voluntary auspices, often a church. A board of directors or trustees, made up of community business, professional, and religious leaders, are the so-called dollar-a-year people (if that) with a paid, full-time administrator and small operating staff.

There are Richter-size rumbles in Washington that are shaking the voluntaries. Congress has threatened to examine their nonprofit ratings to see whether the community benefits from that tax-exempt status. The difference between a for-profit and nonprofit has been questioned. The Internal Revenue Service (IRS) is questioning the excessive executive compensations and the corporate pacts between the HMOs and the hospitals. A system that has a for-profit business organization uses an alleged nonprofit arm all under the same blanket. The IRS has not been blind to the business arrangements between the institutions and their corporate parents. We will wait and see on that one. The business of America is business.

Proprietary hospitals are pure commercial establishments, and they are profit-intending institutions. Or at least they do their darndest to make it that way. They are usually owned by corporate entities and occasionally by a coterie of that hospital's doctors.

Then there are the hospital corporations that usually own a chain of institutions located locally or nationally. They also have added on nursing homes and other types of healthcare facilities that include outpatient clinics and surgical centers. In the U.S., these are becoming medical empires and exert enormous influence through lobbies in Washington that do as much as anyone or anything in deciding the course of healthcare in the nation. They are, of course, staunch protectors of privatization and are getting married up with HMOs and their insurance parents as we speak.

Finally, there are the government-supported hospitals that are totally under the aegis of the federal government with state and local administrations and subjected to local and federal budget restrictions. Their facilities, personnel, and numbers of beds fluctuate depending on those funds year to year. These include all major city hospitals, often without private services or beds but which can be attached in body and spirit to a proprietary hospital wing that uses the same facilities and medical staffs. After all, the medical students and resident staffs have to learn on somebody. How else could they get ready to treat the paying customers? Veterans' hospitals fall into this category but are exclusively federally and publicly financed and administered.

Studies have confirmed the obvious. Proprietaries have a bottom line to meet. Even the AMA, still the protector of the status quo, has published in its journal *(JAMA)* a report of over a half million patient discharge records. The report indicated that while uninsured patients were in less stable medical condition than the privately insured, they were nonetheless discharged sooner. A study from the *Journal of General Internal Medicine* found that patients in for-profit hospitals are up to four times more likely than in the nonprofits to suffer complications from surgery or have delays in diagnosing and treating ailments.

THE VETERANS AND PUBLIC HEALTH

Public and veteran hospitals are subsidized by various statutes. They are suffering, as well. Many of these are married in different ways to local general proprietary and voluntary and university/medical school hospital centers. Their finances are so intertwined that when funds dry up from Washington for those hospitals via Medicaid and Medicare, it curtails much needed medical staff and facilities to the veterans' centers.

A position paper released by the American Public Heath Association (APHA) cautioned the HCFA via Medicaid to at least guarantee continuing full coverage for children as proposed cuts were being scheduled for the rest of the program. APHA's executive director, Georges C. Benjamin, MD, has said that "...public health services...in most cases, have proven to be cost effective...most notably for services like immunizations and post-natal care." These will suffer.

But Dr. Benjamin's words and those of others on his team across the nation are falling on deaf ears. The number of public hospitals in large metropolitan areas declined over the recent years since the end of the 1992 Clinton term and the start of the 2000 Bush II regime.

One hundred major urban centers were surveyed and saw a decline of almost one-fifth of public hospitals. In the suburban areas studied, 27 percent closed. At the same time, as a means of comparison, the so-called proprietary (for-profit) hospitals declined by 11 percent in the cities and 2 percent in the suburbs.

Veterans' hospitals are in the same soup. In the life of just about every living adult in America, the world has not known a single day of total peace. Our own USA has been involved continually with a wartime activity and economy that includes troops from all branches of the armed services. Just do the math.

We sent millions of our guys, and gals, into the Atlantic and Pacific theaters of war from Pearl Harbor to V-E and V-J Days in 1945. Then came Korea in 1951, Vietnam in 1963 for a full decade, land troop skirmishes in Haiti, Panama, Chile, Grenada, Bosnia, Nicaragua, Afghanistan, Iraq I and II (the Desert Storms). The list seems to have no end in sight. President George W. Bush and his cabinet officers, like Secretary of Defense Donald Rumsfeld and Vice-President Dick Cheney, are always quick to warn us that we are in for the long haul when it comes to our soldiers and occupations in far off places. Very far off places. Some many Americans never even heard of.

Gold Star mothers are honored. The vets get to throw out first balls on Opening Day. They get to be Grand Marshall at a July Fourth parade. They even get to sit in an open limo under a storm of ticker tape. They get to have a cup of coffee with a hand shake and photo op in the Oval Office. They get to stroll in the Rose Garden with the president and his cabinet. They get special seats at the party conventions beside the first lady and a nod during the president's speech with a fifteen-second TV sound bite.

What they don't get are assurances of that desperately needed follow-up federal healthcare.

Advice overheard on surgical rounds: Figuring out how to pay your medical bill will keep your mind off your post-op pain. ♦

The Joint Commission (JCAHO)

Accreditation also plays a huge role. The Joint Commission on Accreditation of Healthcare Organizations (JCAHO) has that acronym that puts a scare into the hearts of every hospital administrator. "'Jayco' is coming" is the way it is clamored. Kind of like getting a certified letter "request" from Internal Revenue to pop down to the local IRS office with last year's return.

Billed as a nonprofit commission, JCAHO was formed in 1951 and has become the nation's predominant standards-setting organization, with sponsors from the AMA, The American College of Surgeons, The American Hospital Association, and the American Dental Association, for starters. It is based in Illinois and Washington with about 1,000 people employed in its surveyor force.

Hospital orderlies, house staff, nurses, et al, have to wash the floor, starch their uniforms, and be at work on time when JCAHO comes to town. Up to now, JCAHO visits have been scheduled, but there is a rather well-confirmed rumor that to make things more kosher, those accreditation on-site visitations will come without warning. Generally, 90 percent of hospitals meet JCAHO standards with certain relatively minor failings that must be corrected within a given time period, usually easily met. Less than 5 percent get full accreditation, and another 5 percent will get a stamp of approval but with suggestions that certain services are performing marginally, and those updates are looked at with a sterner eye. Less than 1 percent fail to meet the JCAHO requirements and lose accreditation until corrections are made and approved.

JCAHO's announced goals are like mom and apple pie—improve patient identification, tighten communications between caregivers, assure better safety precautions in general at all levels of care, reduce nosocomial infections, and reduce hospital accidents. For sure, JCAHO's work and motives are well intended. How they all play out in the era of managed care is another side of the story.

As a medical student back in the early 1960s, I was hired on at the Delaware Hospital in Wilmington, Delaware, a community hospital, strictly volunteer, with then a loose teaching arrangement with a medical school in nearby Philadelphia. It was a part of a network with two other similar hospitals in the Wilmington area.

Wilmington, then and now, is home to the Dupont Company, a major player in the field of commercial chemistry, with other arms in the automobile, pharmaceuticals, munitions, rubber, and other industries. It is near the top of the Fortune 500. At the time, the titular head of the Dupont family, Pierre himself, was alive and well and, as was the practice of the entire family conclave, took on particular charities in the city, such as the parks, the symphony orchestra, and holiday fetes. Pierre's pet charity was the healthcare services, and like "Jayco is coming," about every August, he would appear with his entourage, meet with the hospital administration and financial officers, be given a statement for that prior year's expenses, and write out a check for the red ink, usually, at that time, in the neighborhood of about a quarter of a million dollars, even then just petty cash to a conglomerate the size and scope of Dupont, Inc.

On this occasion, however, there was a scare. The budget exceeded the earlier estimate by almost double, and excuses were being prepared by the hospital CEOs with promises to tighten the ship for the coming year. The accounting sheet was presented, and the alibis got underway. There had been a breakdown in the OR and new anesthesia machines were needed, a renal dialysis department was created, and several new EKGs and an X-ray unit were purchased, all unexpected.

It was also noted that the hospital's practice of having a coffee and soft drink station at each of the nine doctors' stations, the surgical suite, and the labor and delivery unit had an overage from the allowed $4,000 to $6,500. Delaware Hospital's president started his apology and pledge to close down this frivolity and stay within budget the following year.

Pierre Dupont held up his open-faced palm and shouted, "Stop!"

He nodded to his assistant to take out the checkbook, write in the full amount, and present it for payment. "Do not close a single way station for the hospital medical staff," he said. "This sounds like a good way for the doctors to relax and get a breather from their demanding routine, and perhaps discuss patient care in a more restful manner." He was handed his hat and cane and walked to the door, promising to meet again in a year, check-book in hand, and wished them his best. ♦

The Healthcare Conglomerates

Managed care and the onslaught of privatization are now setting a new pace. With hospitals picking up the gauntlet of "Silent Cal" Coolidge, they are becoming a part of the business image of the USA—with more than a little help from Washington. Just like their parents, the insurance and banking industries.

There is almost no way to tell how many hospital conglomerates there now are in the country; they are too interwoven and have several interlocking directorates. But just as the managed care insurance companies are gradually filtering down to the handful, what with mergers and acquisitions of their own, the hospital moguls are following suit.

For openers, there is Amerigroup, listed last year in *Forbes* magazine among the twenty-six "best managed companies" in the "health-care equipment and services category" in America. Its arms make any octopus look like Venus de Milo. Its listing includes Aetna, Affiliated Healthcare, Inc., various Blue Cross/Blue Shield (called: Blue Cross/Blue Steal by one healthcare activist group), CIGNA, Humana Inc., Boston Scientific, and WellChoice.

Humana, Inc., a multibillion dollar healthcare behemoth headquartered in Louisville, Kentucky, is by itself one of the nation's largest publicly traded health benefits companies, with approximately 7 million members in fifteen states and services peddled to employers, government-sponsored plans, and individuals. Humana's arms are also octopi in scope, with subsidiaries that are too plentiful to trace. Its net income rose by 60 percent from 2002 to 2003 and 43 percent in 2004.

These healthcare empires, as mentioned above, do get their fair share of Congress' ears. That lobby they maintain is only the tip of the iceberg. Sometimes, they show their oats so hubristically that you might think they'd be embarrassed. No such thing.

Frist Aid

How about having an "owner" of what may be the largest chain of for-profit hospitals in the country avoid the middleman, the lobby, and just put himself right smack dab in the Senate of the United States of America? Wait, there is more. It gets better. Then he gets nominated and elected by his peers as the majority leader, with control over virtually every bill and piece of legislation that gets to the floor for a debate or vote. In fact, unless the majority leader says so, it won't even ever get to that vote or debate. And with every indication that he is seriously considering a run for the presidency. Now that would be something. And that is exactly how it is!

The Healthcare Company (HCA) changed its name in May 2000 from Columbia/HCA Healthcare Corporation in the wake of its tainted image as a part of the largest healthcare fraud ever in U.S. history. Nashville, Tennessee-based HCA runs over 340 hospitals, 135 outpatient surgery centers, and better than 200 nursing homes and home healthcare agencies across the country. It agreed to a fine of $745 million to partly settle a federal investigation into its defrauding the Medicare program. An added settlement figure was awaiting a final tally by the HCFA.

HCA was the original name of the company founded by the Tennessee Frist family in 1968. In 1994, Columbia, another healthcare giant, acquired HCA for $7.5 billion. Some of the allegations by Medicare stemmed from before that acquisition.

The head HCA honcho was one Thomas Frist, Sr. Second in command was his number one heir, Tom Junior, and guess who was numero duo—no one other than Republican Majority Leader Bill Frist, M. D. Yes, that Bill Frist. With pun intended, one political reporter called this set up Frist Aid.

Patricia Frist, Bill's sister-in-law, was also politically attached to the right people and the healthcare industry. She was a one-woman lobby in her own right, spending lavishly over the years. She made the *Mother Jones* top 400 contributor list consistently by giving over $100,000 in soft money to the GOP national committee. HCA kicked in almost $400,000 for the 1996 campaigns, plus individual family members adding to the swill. And whereas Tom Senior and Junior have an array of other financial interests, Bill has more or less confined his portfolio to healthcare equities, once reporting a personal fortune of about $20 million, well better than half of which was in HCA stock. His financial well-being depends strictly on the HCA bottom line. Talk about special interests!

So what has been happening in the Senate these past few years? Frist is the outspoken advocate for Medicare options, meaning having the managed care wings get more and more power and more and more federal reimbursements for each Medicare recipient enrolled. For starters, he teamed up with West Virginia Democrat and another first-family scion, Senator Jay Rockefeller. Together, they managed to enable provider-sponsored organizations to compete with the HMOs for Medicare patients. HCA's profits from these transactions can only be called tidy. Enough said.

Dr. Frist has even gone up against the White House when it comes to touching the healthcare dollar, although that issue is neither clear or without suspect. Bill Frist has certainly toed the mark every other time for his party hierarchy. When Bush and VP Cheney, et al, have told Dr. Frist to jump, he asks how high. There was a hand-me-down from the Oval Office recently that was going to result in a reduction in patient reimbursements to the Medicare HMOs by over $5 billion. At a billion a day needed for Iraq, something had to give. When that eventually filtered down to hospital accounts receivable, a Frist Aid pinch would have been heard around the world. This was a result of an accounting office audit that found at least a governmental 5 percent overpayment. Frist stated that might be a good thing. "(the excess)... will attract more managed care companies into the market and drive prices down."

Now, you might think that such an apparent conflict of interests would have raised some eyebrows. It has in the past, with many a public servant at least going through the motions of "divesting of any conflicting interests" or putting things in a "blind trust," as though that made a difference in what follows. But it does look and sound good to the constituency. Bill Frist didn't even bother to do that. Talk about hubris! He stated, more than once, "Sure, it could become an issue. ...There is a stone wall that comes between any [PAC] money that I get...and what I do here." The heat got too much to bear, however. In late 2005, Senator Frist, likely looking ahead to that possible Oval Office campaign, went the blind trust route.

Hospitals have been caught in a vise. They depend on reimbursements from third-party payers, like insurance companies and the HMO complexes, and of course from Medicare and Medicaid, without which just about no hospital could exist. You could count the survivors on one hand. There have been many tricks of the trade in order to make it. Hospitals continually try to negotiate with the carriers in order to get upgraded from primary to secondary to even tertiary. Or employ other subtle manipulations.

The medical community is well aware of a change in ownership and service that were directly a result of that type of suspect negotiation.

In the mid 1970s, a major urban proprietary hospital and its medical school were on the financial brink. A generation of poor grant allocations from private and governmental sectors had finally taken its toll. The fancy corporate CEO board of directors just didn't do its job. It had to close up shop and move to a lower rent neighborhood in the suburbs. That was the easy part. That was even all available. What to do with the hospital structure with its prime real estate and facilities was another story.

The problem was solved with a bit of legerdemain. It seems that a local church group, well connected with the state administration and the governor's mansion, cut a deal. The church machinery, although it probably might have even raised the necessary financing legitimately, was hoping to set up the soon-to-be abandoned hospital complex as a chronic disease rehab center for children, a worthy cause if ever there were one. But to make the dollars work, it was arranged to have the new hospital center become rated as a tertiary unit, with Medicare, Medicaid, and all other carriers from managed care that follow their leaders play the same game. It was a strict political quid pro quo. Future favors were a part of the handshake.

Thus, the property and facilities were dealt away, the reimbursements took care of the sale price, and the taxpayers ended up footing the bill, without even realizing it or even knowing about it, handing over a very lucrative property and buildings to the church—just about free of charge. The property remained off the tax books, so no commercial value was ever derived for John Q. Public. The church group took in the profits. Another case closed. ♦

Although the Frist family and their entrepreneurial talents may be at the top because of their humongous numbers, don't think they are the only ones in the medical family who are taking advantage of business being the business of America. Too many have crossed the line in the HMO/Hospital v Doctor/Patient lineup. These rebellious doctors, seeking new ways to turn a buck in this era of falling reimbursements and obeying the old adage of if you can't beat 'em, join 'em, actually end up pitting themselves against their medical colleagues.

They end up controlling their pals' shoestrings. Some have gone as far as building new hospital units in many of the popular specialties and then sending referral patients on to those institutions in direct competition to the hospitals where they are staffed. It has gotten to the point where hospitals, while having their doctors fill out long-winded application forms for staff privileges, demand to know if the doctors are involved in any fiduciary or fiscal way with other medical centers. They can try then to deny them staff privileges.

But by far, the majority of the U.S. medical community has preferred to live by an old aphorism often heard in doctors' dining rooms—"a business person I am not." Physicians have notoriously been teased for becoming the "suckers" in many a business shuffle, just never willing or able to spend the time and energy on such matters. The demands made of them in general in their medical routines are so excessive there is just no time for anything else.

Paddy Chayefsky's 1971 historical full-length sardonic movie, "The Hospital," was a little before its time. In an exaggeration to make a point (but not much of an exaggeration, for I have known true doctor characters like them) Chayefsky had one doctor character talk business and stocks and property and what have you on the phone with his broker during patient bedside visits and spend his time during staff conferences badgering his colleagues into one business deal after the other. The doctors' defense almost always includes the adage that competition makes for higher-quality patient care. To many on the outside and in Paddy Chayefsky's audience, it was discomforting to watch as their lives and limbs depended on their physicians' business acumen rather than medical skills. What looked like such a hyperbolic caricature then seems more in sync today. Perhaps even tycoon Pierre Dupont would have squirmed if his staff were using their coffee klatches to discuss their stock portfolios rather than patient pre- and post-op needs and complaints. ♦

How exactly hospitals are reimbursed by either the third-party commercial carriers or the government out of Washington, and the funds filtered down through the various respective state capitals, could and would be explained five different ways by four so-called experts. The system seems so complicated and convoluted that hospital financial officers are content not to understand the whole process but rather settle for their own bottom lines month to month and just hope they come out in the black.

Although the reimbursements are, in the end, based on those primary, secondary, or tertiary labels, that in itself relies on yet other means of determination. For example, there is the Graduate Medical Education (GME) rating, which may indeed be the basis for it all. The GME is the administrative arm of the system that decides the hospital's worth in facilities, staff skills, and training and a general ability to deliver teaching and patient care. The number of residents-in-training is assigned to each hospital and in each of the specialties accordingly.

Obviously, the more residents, the higher the quality of the hospital and the wider the scope of its facilities. An accredited hospital with an array of residents that numbers in the many hundreds, plus the space, equipment, and personnel on all levels to, say, perform cardiac transplants, would be issued tertiary status automatically. A hospital with a handful of residents and dependent on its voluntary staff for its twenty-four-hour-a-day coverage and allowed, say, normal deliveries and cardiac stabilization before shipping the patient to a cardiac center, would be assigned primary, or community, status. The secondary status is somewhere in between.

It was in 1964 that I started my residency training in my gynecological specialty at a major Eastern city medical school training center. I was paid $200 a month, net. There were neither FICA (Social Security), any income taxes, nor Medicare contributions deducted, if they applied. It was explained that the house staff was being classified and paid as students, and therefore none of the above applied. That had been the hospital's policy and practice for many years.

About halfway through my training years, what had been battled in court without my knowledge came to a decision. Apparently, the federal accountants and attorneys had successfully argued that house officers were not students but employees of the hospital and the government treasury was entitled to such payments. After a perfunctory appeal, the red-faced hospital made a settlement *to cover the monies due the Treasury Department and our future paychecks were reflective. The hospital CPAs computed how much we would have to be paid to net out at the $200 figure. As it came out, I was thereafter paid $200.18 per month. I felt like I got a raise.* ♦

Hospital CFOs

The eventual reimbursement from all sources takes into consideration what is labeled direct payment, meaning the actual salaries paid the residents on staff, and the indirect allowances, consisting of the ancillary funds needed for such things as meals, uniforms, medical library books and equipment, sleeping facilities, and the like.

They are also based on an entity called the Case Mix Index (CMI), which figures into the primary, secondary, or tertiary status given. Since Medicare has adopted a DRG rating system for compensation to assuage the staunch complaint that dumping and the other practices could make it an uneven playing field, a system was inaugurated to blend in the cases and the extent of the treatments needed based on a period of previous experience. This vain attempt to account for the inequities of the DRG method is put into the equation to set a hospital's rating.

There are then the human elements that perhaps are the most important factors of all. Ego and negotiations.

Hospital CEOs, CFOs, and department chairs spend a good deal of their time in debate and negotiations with the federal people, and subsequently, the insurance carriers and their HMOs, to set a rate at which the hospital will get paid. That alone is enough to account for the line up that has put the hospitals and their paymasters, the HMOs, on one side of the tug-of-war and the loyal doctors and their patients on the other.

The importance of keeping the beds filled, the turnover based on DRGs and the CMIs and efficient use of equipment and facilities are primordial when crunch time comes about. JCAHO makes its regular visit, and the HMO financial wizards come in to determine how much the hospital will get for each bed occupied per day, the number of sonograms performed and why, the operating room efficiencies, and monthly costs.

The days of sugar daddies like the Dupont brothers and the few others are long gone. The complexities of medical life and times in the USA, with its multipayers and bureaucracy, have created the competition that Bill Frist predicted. But, it has not filtered down into lower costs for the patient. The price of that bureaucracy is three times or more than any other country with a national health service, which, I remind you, is everybody else.

At one major city medical school hospital center, the internationally respected chair of obstetrics and gynecology, after fifteen years of service and still in relative youth and energy, offered his resignation. To the shock and dismay of the board of directors, and upon learning that money and pension perks were not the issues, the board was given an explanation it could not correct. The chair informed the board that he would stay on for another term if he were appointed co-chair, with his other half given the responsibility of approving the color of curtains, vacation schedules for secretaries, and most of all, those boring and tedious negotiation sessions with the HMOs for rates and allowances for patient care. All he wanted to do was clinical and research medicine, not administrative duties. And he also asked he be excused of what, in a single word, had become the scourge of every hospital chair—meetings. "Meetings just to schedule meetings," was the way he put it. Needless to say, the board declined and formed a search committee (read: more meetings) to select a more pliable replacement. ♦

Tertiary teaching hospitals, with a full resident complement, are not faring any better than their lower-ranked counterparts in striving for better payment rates.

Competitive market pressures have caused many teaching programs to either curtail their individual specialty training or cut back to bare minimums. Dr. David Blumenthal, a director of services at the prestigious Massachusetts General Hospital in Boston that is a part of the Harvard network, has said, "If this [hospital] were in the business community, you would see [some] of these institutions filing for bankruptcy."

Nursing schools have been closed and research pursuits for new technologies have felt the sting. Reports are creeping into the literature that are urging Medicare and other federal funding sources to stop the cutbacks planned for the years ahead. But the HMOs and the insurance people have turned away their ears and eyes.

Hospital Occupancy Rates & Turnover: Time is Money

One of the most apparent ways the HMO/managed care entity is showing its cost-cutting shenanigans is starting with finding ways, any ways, of cutting down hospital inpatient stays.

Author Barbara Gordon in *I'm Dancing As Fast As I Can* explains her title with a vignette about a couple on the night club floor at a hotel singles weekend. "I'm only here for the weekend," the gentleman says. She replies, "I'm dancing as fast as I can."

As hospitals in this age of managed care HMO-style are taking hold, trying to get people out the door in a hurry, the patients could be saying, "We are healing as fast as we can."

What I went through with Jessica Riggins is being experienced by many of my colleagues as a routine. Those in obstetrics were the first to live with that change in practice. In the era of my residency training, a four- to five-day post-partum hospital stay was the routine. A day or two more after cesareans. Those countries with their forms of a national health service even kept their parturients for a full week. There were valued post-delivery classes for breast feeding and new baby care. Studies showed how much this rest and rehab were so appreciated by the patients preparing for their new adventures into motherhood.

Managed care has changed all that. First it was with normal deliveries, then to cesareans. Twenty-four-hour stays have become the new practice. If that long. An added overnight for the post-cesarean is permitted—sometimes. Just as with Jessica Riggins, it is based on the hour of the day you were admitted and delivered. "Revolving-door obstetrics" is the way it became known. The metaphor fits.

It soon spread to other surgical procedures and was immediately carried to an extreme, as the Jessica Riggins saga described. The problem was not that easy to deal with and debate because there were indeed many instances when some patients and some procedures were better managed at home or halfway houses or the system was abused. But those were the exceptions. The driving inspiration behind the dramatic reductions in hospital stays, without doubt, has been fiscal. Profits before people.

Often, doctors will discharge their patients at an earlier time than preferred only because the trouble and paperwork and phone calls and explaining (as I did with Jessica Riggins) just becomes too time-consuming and aggravating. Instead, they cross their fingers and hope for the best. Then, when they get away with it every so often, they get in the revolving door habit. A dangerous one.

Comparisons have been made with those other industrialized nations with their national health services, where hospital stays are not a factor. Indeed, Germany, England, and Canada, for example, with their more generous lengths of inpatient stays than the U.S., still have their lower relative healthcare costs. Their U5MRs are under ours. There has to be a cause and effect.

Another fallout to that shorter stay philosophy has the doctors using varieties of medications for both the healing process and analgesia only with that discharge in mind.

The clinicians often must come to a decision, deep in their thinking, that they will withhold certain narcotics or other medications that demand a closer scrutiny, either because of their toxic profile or their relative newness to the market. The doctors will opt—or should I say, have to opt—for a management and medication that is older, with a more extensive history and a known profile. If the patients were to remain as inpatients, other drugs might have been preferred. The doctors are at the horn of a dilemma. Their loyalty is to the patients. Their monthly profile sheet is with the hospital and its managed care overseer.

And profiles are what they are called. Drill sergeants and reprimand sheets are what they are. They are first-class evidence as to where the final sides have been drawn. For although the doctors and their hospitals once had a family-oriented relationship with only one combined goal in mind—the care given to the patient through a quality hospital—they have now taken a 179 degree turn.

Each month, generated by a master computer somewhere in the bowels of the hospital administration office, every staff physician gets a printout of his/her past month's experience with anything that involves the use of hospital facilities and services. The sheets include each patient visitation, the dates of admission and discharge, the days as a patient, and operating and recovery time if they apply. Then, to put the fear of retribution in the clinician's mind, there are those tabulations of the patients' experiences and then a comparison number matching those figures against the doctor's peers, colleagues, and other staff members. The message is clear.

The doctors are being looked upon as bad team members if they go above and beyond the average. Marking them as those who do not have the quality of skill and medical acumen to match their peers. The immediate tendency is to scream that no such comparisons are valid; how can you juxtapose one doctor against another when you are not accounting for the patients' histories, pathologies, and hospital needs?

Nor are you looking at the physicians' training and possible postgraduate fellowships and programs that have given a particular clinician the expertise to take on more perilous cases that inevitably face a greater morbidity and mortality. Instead, the assumption is that you are merely being stacked up against a similar group from a like catchment area of patients, and thus, in the long run, the pathology and needs will average out. And maybe that is true to some extent. By the demographics, that is logical. But not in practice.

The physicians are made to feel apologetic, even ashamed that they haven't matched up to standard. If they persist in those numbers that are considered aberrant, they are called "into the principal's office" to account for their performances that have been deemed at least not in the flow by the hospital administration, acting as obvious flunkies for its HMO/managed care supervisor. There have been many staffers with a lengthy tenure and in good standing who have been earmarked for not playing under the new rules and get placed on probation.

There are those who have indeed been reprimanded to the point of having their hospital privileges suspended until they get with the program. When the doctors seek redress and get together with the hospital medical board and administration, all on a first-name basis, they are sadly informed of the new set-up and instructed to get on board. I leave it to your wonderment if that sort of peril does not influence how the doctors' upcoming patients are treated and discharged the next time around.

A few years ago, I was called into federal court in Los Angeles to testify on behalf of a group of Mexican-American women who, upon seeking help from the LA County Hospital for their perceived infertility, were informed that at their last delivery, all eventually done by cesarean section, their fallopian tubes had been ligated, resulting in permanent contraception. The defense by the University of Southern California medical school service included that these women had duly signed informed consents, properly translated into their native Spanish. These women were all of strict Catholic faith, wherein such a practice was highly frowned upon.

It was then revealed, and not denied by the defendants, that the signings had indeed been scribbled on the forms—during the heights of their labors.

I presented to the court more than a full day's testimony in the dock that under the stress of labor pain, or any pain for that matter, when patient thinking and the decision process would have been distorted, "informed consent" was an oxymoron and therefore invalid. This thinking had then and since been accepted by virtually every medical center and obstetric authority in the country. So-called "informed consents" are no longer permitted during the labor process. What's more, since that hearing in LA, the federal government, in all publicly financed services such as under Medicare, Medicaid, and the armed forces, requires that a consent for a tubal ligation be agreed to in writing twice. First, at least thirty days prior to the expected day of confinement, and second, at the time of the proposed surgery, as a way of further assuring the consent was truly informed, emphasizing the electivity of the procedure and its permanence. That regulation became a welcome standard for all cases, private and service, in the city of New York. Other cities with independent medical machinery from their states are considering following suit.

In court, however, my several hours of grueling testimony were dismissed as unacceptable with a single sentence in a thirty-page decision by the presiding judge in a nonjury trial as "some doctor from New York" (I was not mentioned by name, although other witnesses were) who ruled in favor of the medical center. There were no funds available to mount an appeal. ♦

Who Watches the Watchdogs?

The insurance company/HMO gatekeepers are now hiring gatekeepers for the gatekeepers. I have seen the documentation from several colleagues of letters received from their HMO units that have indicated that after a review of the clinician's treatment over that past several years for hundreds of patients, some have been rejected as excessive or unacceptable. This, to practitioners who are considered at the vanguard in their fields of specialty. The HMO thus requested a refund of a portion of the fees paid to the doctor and ordained that his/her practice be altered to comply with the updated HMO standards of care. All known such cases to date have been for office procedures and care. Hospitals that had already negotiated a reimbursement rate have not been subject to this type of review. Which means all hospitals.

Negotiations have been the rule of the day over these many years. No two patients are alike; no two managements are alike; no two doctors are alike. Physicians in the exact same specialty with the same procedural and billing codes have bargained for different rates of reimbursement by the carriers. What this all depends on remains something of a mystery. Since the procedures are essentially the same, this is likely based on volume, location, exclusivity of practice, and just good salesmanship on the part of the physician.

Hospitals have done exactly the same. Hospital CEOs and their financial wizards sit down over cocktails and dinner and hammer out "a deal." They base their deal, of course, on the number of usable beds; the facilities; whether the unit is primary, secondary, or tertiary; the hospital's track record of success; the reputation of the staff; and the financial strength of the hospital board.

That is where the utility of the hospital comes in. That is where the occupation rate plays a role. That is what is behind the "revolving door" hospital turnover. And the negotiations begin. Once the hospital and HMO have set a number, the hospital has to deliver the doctors, the procedures, and the occupation and turnover rates. That revolving door spins a bit faster.

Hospitals Walk Down the Aisle and Stand at the Alter

Such negotiations are behind the many mergers and acquisitions that are becoming commonplace in the American health scene. In New

York City alone, as just one example, four hospital behemoths became two in the past several years. New York Hospital (Cornell University) and Presbyterian Hospital (Columbia University) have become New York Presbyterian. Their medical schools, with their separate boards, have stayed out of the marriage contract. Their prenuptial agreements were specific on that point. The rivalry between medical schools, their department chairpersons and deans, and their individual reputations are just too strong to bargain away. University Hospital (New York University) and Mount Sinai Hospital (City University of New York) also took their vows and became one. On the West Coast, the University of California and Stanford University Hospitals in San Francisco joined teaching and clinical facilities. Others around the country are following suit.

The reasons behind these mergers could make good fiscal sense when the smoke and mirrors are cleared away. The HMO managed care moguls say that by combining their forces and facilities, even as ubiquitous and productive as they were before the mating, the unified medical service organization becomes much more efficient in delivery of services. The feds through the National Institute of Health (NIH) and Congress have adopted this practice, as well, and perhaps there are some advantages. Their grants are reflective.

When the NIH, for example, awards a grant to a particular center and a similar one to a second research lab, they are both told that if they unify their units, the endowment would be more than doubled for those very reasons. Could be.

On occasion, there are personal scrapes and confrontations because one or the other hospital has an invested interest in a service, but the other does not want to give up its own that had been in competition. These things have to be compromised before the deal is signed. But when the HMOs and their carriers and the NIH speak with the big bucks, compromises are somehow always found.

The stand-off between the staff doctors and even their own hospital administrators can get in the way. The administrators then come to wear two hats—one as a practicing clinician on occasion, and the other as the financial and administrative officer. That newly combined New York Presbyterian awarded its president and CEO over $3 million in annual salary and benefits. Others on his office staff take home similar paychecks. They are not the only ones. All part of the overhead.

This reminds me of the oft-repeated gag about the time when baseball superhero Babe Ruth was given a 1928 contract for $100,000, setting a new record for a pro athlete at the time. When he was chided that he was paid more than the president of the United States, that very same Cal "The business of America is business" Coolidge, the Babe replied, "Why not? I had a better year." ♦

The EMR: Who Benefits?

The electronic medical record (EMR) is fast finding its way into hospital and doctor offices for more than their accounts payable and receivable. Patient records are becoming computerized. My own hospitals are on their way. A departmental staff meeting starts with the announcement that on a certain date, usually just a few short weeks ahead, there will no longer "be any such thing as a paper record." Every event, every nursing and medication order, and every nursing and physician progress note will from that moment on be created onscreen or, if by a pen onto a paper chart sheet, scanned that night onto a computer disk. The chart becomes a permanent software record and only the computer literate, allegedly with HIPAA permission, of course, will be able to access it for study and use.

And, like waiting to learn metrics, the changeover is not sitting around waiting for "the old people to die." They either get with the program or move out of the way.

The hospital spokesperson is quick to do a not-so-soft sell on a skeptical staff that is being told of a *fait accompli*. The EMR, it is announced, will be the new and efficient way to go. No longer will nurses have to rush through mounds of charts and piles of papers to find notes, lab results, and appointment schedules. It is just a matter of learning which buttons to touch on the keyboard.

An official Health and Human Services Department report is quoted that expects a savings of billions from our trillion dollar healthcare expenditures just by going "with the program."

Spyros Andreopolis, the emeritus director of public affairs at the Stanford University School of Medicine in California, has tried to put this thinking in the context of the nation's managed care system, further exposing the true role of the EMR.

No one can deny its potential advantages. The EMR will eventually make it easier to follow disease patterns in patients and instantly bring up evidence-based medical data to be a guide to treatment. Or it will flash an array of potential side effects of a considered medication and prevent redundant and unnecessary lab tests and diagnostic procedures. And not while some secretary or departmental clerk will be frantically searching for missing documents or misplaced records, especially from another hospital or office many miles away. It would all be done at the speed of fiber optics, over the Internet, or at a pace set by telephone lines, or satellites in space.

However, the opportunities for misuse will loom greater than ever. Those with a modicum of computer skills will be able to use cyberspace as though they were listening in on the hospital or doctor's office extension line. Employers can screen the undesireds and reject candidates based on personal prejudices. Insurance carriers will be able to touch a tab key and uncover preexisting conditions that would otherwise not be permitted to exclude an applicant from needed coverage. Big Pharma is already exploring ways of using such data to detect a glitch in the patient's medical history and peddle medical services and drugs. It seems like a complete contradiction to what HIPAA was supposed to guard against. And with HIPAA's loopholes that ease the way for the HMOs to gain information legally, no one is quite sure where this will be taken.

Going electronic in this way is certainly an example of IM MacDonald's adage that the only difference between men and boys is the price of their toys. $E=MC^2$ has changed everything. Hospitals have become prey to those new toys out there.

But aren't we forgetting something? Since the purpose of a healthcare apparatus is taking care of people who are sick and want to get better, have any of those alleged savings by the EMR toys filtered down into doing just that? That is not a rhetorical question.

In this age of electronic billing and coding, hospitals are finding out that a more system-savvy clerk can increase their reimbursements by working with the coding systems and nothing more. Just as, for example, General Motors makes a greater return by its money manipulations than by making a better car on a more efficient assembly line, hospitals are discovering the same advantages. A coding-legerdemain of the DRGs by a computer maven can prove to be quite rewarding.

Different diagnosis codes have been assigned different billing codes for the computer, and the electronic experts in the hospital accounts receivable office have learned to manipulate those numbers, outline the procedures in a different lineup, and change the principal to secondary diagnoses to augment the HMO returns. Nothing to do with patient care; only depends on financial jockeying. The business of hospitals is business.

Community, or primary, hospitals receive patient care revenue from the same variety of sources as all others, although on a simpler level because their services are so much less sophisticated. Medicare and Medicaid do account for financial support to the nation's hospitals, without which they could not survive. The commercial insurers, after that negotiation process, then come on board in either a fee-for-service or a negotiated per diem or capitation.

The primaries have often experienced discrimination from their payment sources and have been generally demoted in the eyes and payouts of the carriers. They have, therefore, worked to upgrade the DRG allowances. The feds tend to augment the more intricate DRGs, and the lower-range DRGs suffer, sometimes even with a decrease in payment.

The paymasters argue that the primaries are worth that much less because their care level is well below the "expensive" tertiary kind, and primaries' overheads should reflect that, as well.

The American Academy of Family Physicians (AAFP) has an ongoing study that so far has examined 37 million patient records. The AAFP reported that the lower-end hospitals in the years 2001–'03 had a significantly lower number of patient safety accidents, 20 percent fewer infections, and a statistically significantly fewer nosocomial deaths. In addition, after the first year's report, the upper echelon tertiaries showed a greater improvement than the lower end.

The answer for many has been if you can't beat 'em, join 'em. In the Pittsburgh area, a community hospital had been competing directly with the city's tertiary center for cardiac catheter lab patients. The two had developed a working affiliation, and both seemed to thrive. However, the university center suddenly severed that arrangement. A CFO had determined this made better fiscal sense. The battle lines were drawn.

Many of the doctors were dually staffed and succumbed to the pressures exerted by the university center to use its catheter lab and enjoy the benefits of having the various other high-range services available. The primary boards got some revenge by setting up their own community alliance. It was touch and go for a while. Then came the bottom line. The HMOs and their carriers obviously offered a better reimbursement rate to the tertiary center and were willing to coattail the communities if they became subservient to their tertiary bosses. The hospital staffs wondered loud and clear why they were at odds with their own administration. They had forgotten the business of America is business. ♦

"Frist aid" stated that competition among the hospitals resulted in better patient care. Again, when treatments are dictated by MBAs instead of MDs who have held up their right hands and taken the Oath, their goals are quite different and they act accordingly.

A university faculty poll analyzed 341 HMO plans operating in various markets throughout the U.S. Their results were not all that surprising to those who knew the score from the very start. Although the good ol' definition of competition in an open market has been a capital-oriented goal in order to lower prices, that does not seem to filter down when healthcare is involved. HMO competition was centered about the plans' premiums, with little attention paid to healthcare quality. Surprise!

In comparison to other industries, say, the highly competitive automotive, elements such as emissions, fuel efficiency, and safety measures are regulated. With hospitals, pharmaceuticals, for example, a major cost issue, are not. Some of the proprietary hospitals would not report their data, and thus, many conclusions were never drawn. But it is suspicious that they had to be hiding something. The researchers did add that the healthcare environment is complicated and multilayered. So more time and more study are needed to finalize the so-far damaging conclusions.

There have been some indications that doctors' groups have made threatening moves against the HMOs and even the hospitals that stand between them as a buffer. Doctors now seem willing to go up against their HMOs; they do have second thoughts about their hospitals. They once considered them their family. At one time, a federal court ruled vaguely that physicians' suits against their HMOs were not admissible. Then a Miami district federal judge wrote that such suits challenging HMO business practices could move forward.

But the plaintiffs' claim that the HMOs had acted in violation of the Racketeer Influenced and Corrupt Organizations (RICO) act was dismissed by the same court. So, although the suits are moving ahead, both sides have already claimed a victory. Such litigation is cropping up all over the place. Doctor groups are even suing their HMOs for their slow payment and for suddenly reducing reimbursement rates. The problem is that—like all insurance carriers—HMOs are in a no-lose situation. If the decision should ever go against them, demanding faster and more dependable payments to their providers, they will simply react by raising premiums on their clients. So their profit/loss statements will remain intact.

This accentuates how starkly the sides have been drawn. Doctors go to work every day for their HMO bosses, whom they consider their antagonists. They work for them one day and "take them to court" the next. The system all seems so convoluted.

So what has all of this meant to hospitals, their staffs, and their commitments to serve the people of their catchment areas? When doctors and the HMOs get into a heavy diatribe, like the Jessica Riggins debacle and worse, when the patients involved do not have the finances and strengths to battle their own HMOs, the doctors are left out on a virtual limb without their patients at their legal sides. That was the significance of the Jessica Riggins victory.

The 2001 Ted Kennedy (D-MA) bill, passed in the Senate with the help of John McCain (R-AZ), provided legal machinery for patients to take action against their own HMOs, if they were acting against patients and their doctors. The Oval Office opposed the legislation, insisting it would "drive up premium costs and cause many Americans to lose their health insurance." As though it were affordable now.

Some authorities are even wishing for such a thing. They suggest, with some merit, that as the HMOs inflict their pain, as medical activist Kip Sullivan has written, through premium increases, this would be a highly visible irritation to many people. The HMOs maintain their balance sheets in a way that becomes apparent to their victim patients/clients. Managed care either raises the fees or erodes the services.

Just as the pharmaceuticals have always claimed they need their voracious markups on their drug products to cover the costs of those failed medications and their R & D, the HMOs and their hospital clients purport that they need the cushion of profit to provide the array of free care through their services to the poor, especially in their emergency rooms that often have to provide life-saving procedures. There are sick jokes that depict ER clerks getting a financial statement from the patient on one side of the litter while the cardiac resuscitation team is scurrying about trying to insert a life-saving intravenous on the other. A bit of an extreme to make a point, but a point well taken.

Major prestigious medical centers throughout the country are looking for "Frist aid" by bringing HMOs and for-profit hospital chains to the bargaining table. Or closing services. Almost none seem to be impervious. Deaconess Beth Israel Hospital in Boston, a part of the Harvard complex, and the famous Hospital of the University of Pennsylvania in Philadelphia (HUP) have also stirred the waters in that they are dickering with selling their teaching hospitals to a for-profit conglomerate. Tulane Hospital in New Orleans and George Washington University Hospital in the nation's capital have already done so. Many others throughout the country are looking at their enormous debt and, facing staggering deficits, are looking to bail themselves out by selling to those private systems.

As noted, these institutions have kept their medical schools out of the loop. The schools enjoy large philanthropic donations from organizations, wealthy alumni, corporate handouts, and federal National Institutes of Health grants. Not so for the hospitals, which remain separate fiscal entities.

All this did not happen yesterday. It started during the Great Depression and, with minor peaks and troughs since, has been steadily going downhill. Slashes in the Medicare program by just about every administration since its inception have certainly not helped. And even the most renowned centers with international reputations are not secure.

The Emergency Room

Other misconceptions abound. Dangerous ones. For the needy.

One accepted by many is that our hospitals are always there for the poor and the uninsured. Many a doctor, whom you would think would know better, insists that those tens of millions without health coverage "can come to my hospital any time and get the best care in the world. Bring 'em on." The quality of care in our two-tier system is yet another matter. First, that any care at all is accessible is primary.

Hospital emergency rooms (ERs) have always been glamorized by occasional media specials and cinema that won their share of Emmys. Doctor Kildare and Marcus Welby, MD, were from an era or two ago as legacies of those Norman Rockwell images. Now the heroes and heroines don't even get names. They are just from the "ER." Or "911."

White-frocked, unshaven, sleep-deprived and bleary-eyed, haggard-looking emergency room staffers run about stopping massive hemorrhages, saving lives from various traumas, assuaging emotional upheaval, salvaging marriages and broken families, or curing whatever else comes along in myriads of patients—and become matinee idols.

They have, though, since the introduction of managed care, seemingly drawn and enjoyed even more TV sitcom and drama attention. In the present managed care echelon, it is almost as though this is a scheme staged by the PR people to glorify the ER staff physicians to even greater heights in a form of stroking. But, in reality, HMOs are making sure they are kept in their places as HMO "providers."

ERs often represent the first line of care for the indigent, if only out of desperation. Many a crowded waiting area is filled with sniffles, tension headaches, and painful menstrual periods; the patients are aware they have no other access to care elsewhere.

Triage personnel are forever struggling with the patient load, mindful of their duty to allocate need on a priority basis. Many of the admitting clerks are from the neighborhood and identify with the clamoring patients and hate to turn them away, even though they know their needs are not life threatening or emergent, the true purpose of an ER. But the staff also knows that the ER does indeed serve as the patients' doctors, and so they make all sorts of excuses.

In recent years, the most sought-after residency programs in the country have been in emergency medicine, always filled by aspiring medical students. It is commonplace for many a hospital clinic servicing the hospital-based crowd with Medicaid, Medicare, or perhaps bare, to be the follow-up arm for its needy population, seeing "elective" complaints that were first managed by ER visits the day or week before. Hospitals take pride in providing such care, however ambivalently unnecessary, as a mark of their contributions to the neighborhood. It is a way for the system to remain status quo, insisting that a national health service is not needed. "Look, America takes care of its own."

The ERs and the hospital clinics just about all work on a sliding scale when charges are set for the myriad of uncovered patients. Hospitals boast that no one is ever turned away, but that is not entirely true. Many times, the triage staff, intake social workers, and financial managers do not trust the potential clients. Many patients have stolen or borrowed a friend's or relative's Medicaid or union medical card and gone through the charade of being that person in order to get care. This can get mighty tricky when medical complications arise and the hospital must contact the patient for that follow-up, using the details offered at triage. It comes to be quite a surprise when the call or cable is sent for the patient to respond, and that person does not actually exist. Or not at that address and in that family.

A medical malpractice suit was filed by a patient who had come in for a minor outpatient operation at a neighborhood private clinic using her cousin's "borrowed" union medical card. The patient was accepted in good faith, had the procedure performed, but then had a minor complication. Despite that, she sought out the services of an attorney and instituted an action against the doctor and clinic. When it was discovered that the patient had indeed committed fraud, the private carrier/HMO began a criminal action against the patient and her cousin, suspecting collusion. Needless to say, the two became concerned over the potential fallout and never appeared in court for any of the hearings.

The defense attorneys for the doctor ran into a dilemma. He refused to allow any use of the card switching. The physician reminded the lawyers that he had an ethical and emotional bond with his patient, despite her being at odds with him, because as a doctor sworn in by Hippocrates' Oath, his fidelity was to that patient, no matter how she came to be one. To the doctor, it was not a dilemma; his loyalties were clear. Patient needs were his only goal. The HMO people and lawyers just shook their collective heads in wonderment. ♦

Hospitals have been known to make their own rules when it comes to that sliding scale. After the negotiations are set with the private HMOs and the DRGs and Medicaid fees are handed down by HCFA, the hospitals then use their sliding scale to take care of the rest. And there are plenty of the rest.

The uninsured become the only target left open for grabs. The individual uncovered patients, without the bargaining power of the HMO clientele, are forced into paying "full rates" that the HMO hopes will make up for the negotiated group rates and for those who end up never paying their bills.

And just as patients can sue their carriers for unacceptable medical decisions, the hospitals have been known to sue their patients to recover open invoices. Until it came down to the final stages of her case, Jessica Riggins was threatened with a legal action.

A gentleman patient was being readied for discharge after several days for cardiac stabilization in St. Mary's Hospital Center. As he was collecting his belongings, the Mother Superior head nurse appeared at the door. After a well-wished farewell remark, she asked about the settling up of the bill.

"Do you have any medical coverage?" she asked. "No" came the reply. "How about savings or property in your name?" "Uh-uh." "Are there any friends who can help, perhaps?" "No, not a soul who has that kind of scratch." "How about family?" "Well," he answered, "I do only have one spinster sister left, a little younger, and she is a nun." The head nurse shot back, indignantly, "Sir, your sister is not a spinster. She is married to God." "Oh, fine," he replied. "Then you just send the bill to my brother-in-law." ♦

The Battle Is Heating Up

The hospitals, however, are being challenged. They insist that they only go after those they know are fiscally sound and may even be acting out of deliberate spite and malice. And, in some instances, that is the case. But for the most part, what with the seemingly exorbitant rates of medical care of any quality, it is by far the exception.

It is not unusual for hospitals to go to the trouble of starting collection proceedings against those who extracted needed care as indigents and have absolutely no way of paying such a tab. Why? The hospitals have stated with deliberation that they must act objectively, knowing full well the futility of it all on many an occasion. The message must be delivered that those who can pay must be held responsible or else the hospital legal department will be on their proverbial tails.

The tug o' war between HMO and doctor is not exactly arcane. Hospital bulletin boards are often laden with such postings as "Ten Things Your HMO-Doctor Won't Tell You," which give the clear message that the HMOs can be on one side and the doctors on the other. The HMOs are clearly warning the patients to be careful and not take their doctors too seriously. The HMO is in charge.

And those vignettes about the generalists trying to find specialists are frequent occurrences. A patient's coverage with an HMO will have a primary care internist, for example, based at a certain hospital. But the specialist called for may not be so staffed. The patient either settles for lesser care or moves on. And as we are getting further into the HMO hole, and as more doctors in any given area are HMO-membered, those specialists are harder and harder to find. Physicians who are staying out-of-network and depending on the uncovered or those who are affluent enough to pay the tariff are becoming fewer and farther between.

The HMO is in charge.

Administration after administration, in seeking ways of cutting federal allotments to healthcare, are continually looking to other avenues to cut funds and allotments—after they think the doctors and their institutions have had all they can take for a while.

Nursing homes are where doctors as a group get lined up against their administrations and the HMOs behind it all. Washington always cites fraud and mismanagement as examples of the nursing home extravagances, and every time there is a nursing home owner or board indicted and tried for such abuses, headlines are created by news releases from the White House press room, making sure the public knows of this dalliance. Others abound. We never hear of the cuts made by Medicare, the lifeline of the nursing home industry, or the pinches they are being put through.

"GM" Charlie Wilson said it best. One of the last bastions to hold out against privatization, along with the schools and Social Security, hospitals and the medical community machinery are falling into line.

The commercial nature of hospitals and their services increasingly mirrors the actions and morals of the multinational business world. Corporate mergers and acquisitions are reducing the number of available product sources in every field of commerce. But no business ventures are more threatening to human welfare than those alliances between hospitals and the HMOs. Their intentions should be diametrically opposed, keeping them honest. Instead, they coexist in a parallel universe of shared goals with a mutual enemy—the patient—whose needs and demands hurt their bottom line.

They justify cost-efficient practices at patients' expense. Patient well-being does not enter into their equation. The HMO coyote is guarding the hospital chicken coop.

Big Brother is watching over your hospital dollar, but not necessarily over you. But again, politics makes for strange bedfellows. A new alignment is being formed. On one side are the HMOs and their client hospitals; on the other are the doctors and their patients, right where we all belong. Serendipitously, we finally got it right.

CHAPTER 9

WHY DOCTORS LIE, AND IF THEY DON'T, MAYBE THEY SHOULD

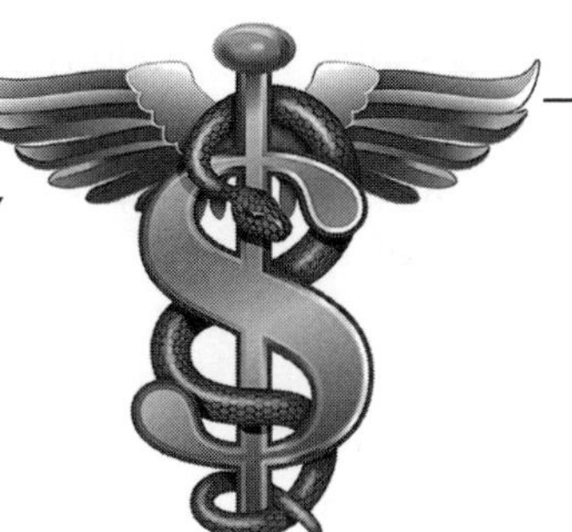

THE OATH OF OFFICE

The Hippocratic Oath that we physicians all take and swear by certainly does demand the *primum non nocere* principle—first, do no harm—as written back in 400 BC by the legendary Greek philosopher well known as the Father of Medicine. Medicine has become an art and practice that today would likely force him to do a little rewrite, or at least some creative editing.

The Oath is sworn to the gods and goddesses, hinting that Hippocrates was not a sexist. It requires and assumes that all physicians stipulate they will teach medicine to the "sons of my teacher" but not to others (nepotism there, wouldn't you say?); practice and prescribe to the best of their abilities; never deliberately do harm *(primum non nocere)* to anyone for anyone else's interest (how about participation in the death penalty?); give "no deadly medicine"; work only for the "benefits of patients"; do nothing beyond the skills the doctor possesses but pass the patient on to those others when needed (the age of specialization); not offer a woman a pessary to produce abortion (shades of Roe v Wade); and not divulge what should be kept a secret (the first HIPAA on record).

The age of modern medicine, when fees and stipulations are very much a part of the game, and where abortion is now the law of the land and doctors participate in legal executions, has made a dent or two in Hippocrates' words. But then again, if the old man knew the reason why some of his philosophies were abandoned, he would likely forgive us all. I think. Don't quote me on that.

But Hippocrates didn't mention verisimilitude. Not a word about the truth; indeed, the words "truth" or "lie" do not appear in the Hippocratic Oath. It is likely that Hippocrates assumed that the doctors of the ancient Greek world would always speak the gospel. Now that we physicians find ourselves either stretching it or outright lying for a variety of reasons, we know, if it is any comfort, that in this one instance, we are not again breaking our commitment.

Perhaps the greatest telltale signature of what has become healthcare in America is that patients count on their physicians to somehow be able and willing to manipulate the mountain of documents, forms, and codes used by the managed care system for billing and reimbursement purposes.

Report after report published by mainstream medical journals, including that of the American Medical Association, describe a pattern of so-called creative invoicing of the HMO so that the doctor can provide the care needed for the patient and also skirt the routine, thus deriving some semblance of financial return that allows the office to stay in business. As the managed care machinery has moved in on medical practices, office overhead has not dropped. In fact, as the yearly cost of living (COL) indices rise, it is still very much a factor. Rent, office property purchases, supplies, office staff wages, and that ever-present bugaboo, medical malpractice premiums, never seem to go anywhere but up. As the physician community takes the hit, it constantly has to negotiate with the HMO carrier, or, as noted, learn to further finesse the billing procedures.

The Billing Codes

Two systems, the International Classification of Diseases (ICD) and the Current Procedural Terminology (CPT) of coding and wording, went into effect worldwide a medical era ago after their introduction by collaboration between the World Health Organization and ten international centers, including one in the United States. The intention was clear and welcome—to promote international comparability of the collection, classification, processing, and presentation of health statistics.

In the U.S., with its privatized *modus operandi,* unique to the entire world, the system took on another role. The two are used as the

CPT and ICD-9 CM (Clinical Modification) for billing purposes. The designation CM has been dropped, so that ICD-9 stands alone. It is updated annually and the new codes, when applicable, go into effect on October first of each year.

The ICD consists of a billing index per diagnosis and contains procedural codes (CPT), which are used for outpatient procedures and inpatient hospital stays and coordinate with the DRG system, née Medicare. The "9" is simply the number of the series so far; ICD-10 is not expected to go into effect until 2007.

These sets of numerical indices have become the household word of every doctor practicing and billing any third-party carrier in the USA In any one specialty, there are literally many hundreds of codes, and eventually, the office staff comes to memorize them out of their constant use and application. There is not a single instance when the billing forms, involving documents or patient submissions to the carrier HMO would not require, as an absolute, both codes. Omitting them is a sure way to an HMO rejection.

The tricks of the trade are now being passed from office to office, and some medical groups and societies have even been bold enough to arrange for public courses and workshops to teach the doctors and their administrative staffs how to use the system to get better reimbursements. That all sounds wise. But, it reads as another battleground between the managed care carriers and the clinician. The plot thickens.

Since their onset, the CPT indices have become more and more elaborate. For instance, there are five levels for a first patient visit, five for an established patient, five others when there is a secondary consult, several for the phone consultations that are sometimes billed and permitted, and finally, there are those categories for what are labeled preventive care. They are based on the time allotted for each patient visit—to the minute. Do not think for a moment that the clinician can automatically use the longest and therefore better-reimbursed CPT. The HMO has built in many safeguards against such a practice. It is a constant tug of war between the doctors' offices and their HMO overseers.

How is the system used? Perhaps it is already obvious. Since that "gatekeeper" is sitting in an office thousands of miles away from the actual doctor and patient, the office staff learns quickly to use creative arithmetic. A sixteen-minute visit becomes twenty or even thirty, and the CPT codes are adjusted accordingly.

A healthy patient visit is invoiced as such. When a type of pathology is discovered that could and perhaps even should be taken care of at that visit, the patient is still requested to return at another time, perhaps a day or so later, and the medical correction is completed. The office can then bill the HMO for that second visit, or a third. This can all be easily justified when the day's office mail included the rental bill, the office maintenance ticket, an ever-increasing utility bill, or more, that ever-looming statement from the malpractice carrier.

The doctor often has to make hard choices. Early retirement? Move to a lower-rent district and chance losing the patient load? Take on an unwanted associate so they can both work on a higher volume? Or simply adjust the ICD and CPT numbers that can get by the carrier.

John was a long-standing friend and med school classmate of mine and had a well-deserved large patient practice in general surgery. My patients had always been pleased with the care John offered. He earned his reputation. We shared several patients over the years.

His office staff was administered by his fiancée, who eventually became Mrs. John. She had been a hospital nurse that we all knew and liked. John's friends and colleagues welcomed their union. Mrs. John ran the show.

When patient Beatrice gave me cause to request a consult with John, I didn't hesitate. My office made the call and appointment. I anticipated the usually satisfactory results.

I was therefore taken aback when Beatrice, a local high school principal and very aware of her health status, came back a few weeks later for her follow-up with me, bitterly complaining of the "care" she received by John's office, particularly from the missus. Beatrice explained immediately, which gave me a sigh of relief, that her anger and refusal to return for John's care was not aimed at him, but at the front office staff.

Mrs. John was going to do Beatrice a "favor." It was explained that Bea was to sign for the office visit and billing forms for the involved HMO, and that she should not become alarmed if the numbers and explanation for the HMO seemed a bit overstated.

Mrs. John was just being resourceful, and with inventive submissions, all true with a bit of a stretch, the HMO carrier would allow more of a reimbursement.

Mrs. John practiced primum non nocere. *Or at least she thought she was. Beatrice's anger was quickly explained. She told me she was very respectful of Doctor John and had appreciated his style and quality of care. But the stretch of the truth got in her way. "If he will allow his office to tell a fib to the insurance company, even on my behalf, he might someday tell one to me."* ♦

Other ploys have become commonplace. Just take two similar patients, with similar or even seemingly identical complaints and demographics. The office time spent with the doctor, the treatments offered and needed, the lab tests carried out, and the follow-up care are alike, too. But read the billing forms sent in to the HMO carrier and it can seem that they were patients with totally different complaints and treatments. When office staff are inventive enough, patients can be listed and their case detailed in such a way that those tacked-on CPTs can multiply the reimbursement rate.

For example, just about all surgical procedures have similar components. The examination of the patient under anesthesia; the insertion of various dyes and medical fluids as diagnostic aids; the opening incision and the surgical machinations that involve various organs that are listed separately instead of as a combined operation. How these are detailed and recorded can often make a difference in how the billing is perceived by the carrier computer.

When surgical procedures are listed in different modes, two identical operations can appear to be quite dissimilar, and the payments by the carrier are, as well. And in this age of electronic technology, when the whole billing process is not even seen or touched by a human eye or hand, a computer program might just let it go by and okay it all.

Sometimes, it is to the great advantage of the surgeon; other times a rejection will be issued, forcing the doctor's accounts receivable to either accept its fate or start the rebuttal process that will require a series of resubmits, and a discussion with the HMO office as I had for Jessica Riggins. All of this adds to the overhead of the insurance company and is eventually passed on to the patient (read: client) in higher premiums.

The HMO never loses. Never.

This is not talking out of school. All of this is common office lore. The carriers are continually on the lookout for such practices. It is not rare for busy clinicians who believe they have, over many years, negotiated and developed an acceptable relationship with the HMO to then find themselves embroiled in an audit, being told that although the billing codes and invoices were approved at the time, the doctor/office is under the suspicion of having exaggerated on those codes or even performing procedures that are now deemed unindicated at a second look at the invoice.

This, despite the patients receiving what they considered excellent and competent care, and continuing their faith in that particular office. Too bad. The HMO decided that the provider acted unnecessarily, the clients had received unapproved and unwarranted care, and a hefty refund is to be paid by the doctor to the insurance company, at risk of being dismissed from its roster as one of its providers.

One AMA study in 2004 (essentially the same results as many others) showed that of over a thousand doctor-patient visits audited, 40 percent of the clinicians had been using one tactic or another consisting of enlarged CPT listings with dramatic ICD diagnoses and embellished patient complaints and symptoms that were near impossible to refute.

When quizzed by the research team under assured anonymity, a quarter of the physicians argued that the payout rate by the HMO was just too insufficient to carry out top-flight care or that without that creativity, the doctors would not have been able to do certain things deemed vital to good treatment but which they knew would have been denied by the carrier HMO.

Phil learned how to play that game not too long after he got started, in his first years as an internist. He had a patient who was denied a certain medication and even a minor procedure by his carrier, and he knew the patient would suffer. The next time around, he bit the bullet, did what he thought best, and charged the HMO accordingly. When it slipped by the gatekeeper and the HMO accounts payable computer, he just made it a practice, many, many times over. He has expressed neither regrets nor guilt. Highway robbery or a fight for survival? Or both? ♦

Were there doctors operating purely out of greed and deception? When their own patients (not "clients") serendipitously benefited? Of course. But by far, the researchers concluded that most of the billing, shamefully admitted as unethical by the many who did it, was a necessary break of ethics. Their patients' needs had been put first, just ahead of the clinicians' own.

Many an observer of the U.S. healthcare system has remarked how degrading it is for physicians to engage in "surreptitious acts of mercy." This is clearly an example of a profit-based, bankrupt medical delivery system that is serving its banking and insurance company masters while forcing their physician providers to resort to deceitfulness. Out of earshot, while still sharing advice and consults about patient medical problems, doctors now compare the many ways they have learned to beat the system. They absolutely consider it a means of survival. And they believe it.

A settlement is now being negotiated out of a lawsuit filed against the Warner-Lambert Drug Company that had been absorbed by Big Pharma member Pfizer. Several years before that takeover, one of W-L's microbiologists blew the whistle on his bosses, claiming he was being asked to ignore federal regulations and help market a drug to physicians for indications for which it was not FDA-approved. It was discovered that Medicaid and other carriers had paid out hundreds of millions of dollars for the medication's distribution to an unsuspecting public, a practice viewed as "experimenting on patients." ♦

"Just-in-case" is the practice of writing out two prescriptions for the patient—the first one truly desired by the doctor to treat the condition, and the other "just in case." Just in case the first one is not on the list of agents allowed for by the HMO, be it Medicaid or a private insurance carrier prescription plan. In a survey by the Kaiser Family Foundation, 2,766 adult women confessed that they went without their needed meds simply because they could not come up with the co-payment at the drug counter.

Diane Rowland, the Kaiser VP who conducted the survey, said, "Even small costs serve as a barrier to care." The study showed that women, with lower incomes than their male counterparts or burdensome responsibilities in one-income families, were more likely to disregard the required medications.

A general practitioner in a northern New Jersey community filed a suit against his HMO carrier following his dismissal from their rolls. This stemmed from an incident that occurred in his office one afternoon when a thirty-five-year-old mother of three staggered into his waiting room complaining of a severe headache and weakness in her legs. The doctor immediately instructed his office nurse to arrange for hospitalization after he evaluated and stabilized the patient. His impression of a relapse of multiple sclerosis proved to be accurate.

However, the insurance company HMO gatekeeper denied the hospital admission until the patient was seen by an HMO neurologist, and the earliest appointment was not until the following day.

"I just dolled up the symptoms and stated she was less responsive than actually true, though not far off. There was no way I would let that lady walk. I guess I am not that good a liar. The HMO staffer caught me in the act and said I was overreacting. I was left almost speechless." ♦

Medical Malpractice: A Unique U.S. Medico-Legal Specialty

Along with being the world's only developed nation without a healthcare plan for its people, as a fallout from a privatized for-profit healthcare system, the USA is also unique in its medical malpractice crisis, yet another reason why American physicians have found it necessary to stretch their imaginations in their management suggestions and reporting.

Fear of litigation from a failed treatment, or an occasional relatively honest misstep that did no meaningful harm, or an innocent unpredictable negative result of treatment has caused many a practitioner to over-dramatize a clinical picture in order to grant their ailing patient tests and analyses that would likely be excessive and unnecessary by the HMO standards and then denied. "Defensive medicine" is what it has been labeled. In mixed company, it is "watch your rear." In doctor-to-doctor bull sessions, it is called by the acronym CYA, "cover your ass."

In contrast, the most severe critics of the national health services in Canada and England are forced to admit that since their advents, "med-mal," as it is known in the trade, is not a factor in those countries. A syllogism has it that if medicine is perceived as Big Business, with the profit and loss of Big Business, then it follows that the ancillary industries that are generated by healthcare delivery should also get into the act. And make a profit. That includes clinical laboratories, the medical supply business, ambulance services, hospitals and...liability insurance (read: med-mal).

The medical malpractice specialty among the nation's lawyers sprung into being, perhaps not coincidentally, with the advent of Medicaid and Medicare in the mid 1960s. For, when we finally created systems that were government run and publicly financed, it followed that private medical insurance programs would be fair game to pay restitution if negligence occurred. Or if it were just suspected.

After all, you sue a plumber if the pipes leak, the contractor if the paint peels, and the auto maker if the bumper falls off. Why not make your doctor accountable for any perceived negligence in care? Makes perfectly good sense. The medical industry is seen, with good merit, as a private enterprise run by entrepreneurs who offer their clients a service by providers. Why not follow the rest of the rules of Big Business and expect compensation if that service or product fails you in any way?

Has it gotten out of hand? Doctors seem to think so. Patients obviously feel that med-mal is justice at work. Malpractice attorneys, now among the leading jurisprudence specialists, are convinced they are doing their clients a valuable service, and of course, in some cases, they are.

But a bevy of attorneys has now sprung up that has given a new meaning to "ambulance chasing." The nation's yellow pages and print and electronic journals are streaked with ads by law offices that ask the public to ponder the potential grounds for a legal action based on their most recent medical care. An untoward pain or ache following surgery? A less-than-desired look after your cosmetic treatment? An infection from a minor office procedure? A bleed you consider excessive? A blur after filling your new eyeglasses prescription? Call your friendly barrister. There may be a big payday in it for both of you.

And with these cases, most often taken on a contingency basis or small retainer, the patients feel they have nothing to lose. That aspect is a major difference between U.S. private healthcare and the NHSs in the United Kingdom and Canada, for example, where contingency fees are not the rule and the patient has to think twice before forking out big bucks to a lawyer on the chance of winning a malpractice action.

Surveys show that half of the actions go no further than an interrogation and review of the records, and jury verdicts are in favor of physician/hospital/defendants about 75 percent of the time. In a few states, defendant physicians and medical facilities triumph as high as 90 percent. I, myself, have reviewed hundreds of possible cases for attorneys regarding potential actions against physicians and have dismissed over 90 percent as being unwarranted from the get go. Fortunately, they then most often go no further. But not always.

There are those attorneys out there who take a case not on its merit but by the physical and personality appeal of the plaintiff or the hunch that they "can make something of it." Med-mal firms have also been known to accept and encourage plaintiff clients because of geography. They come to learn what locations and court districts have more sympathetic jury pools that can turn decisions based solely on emotional conviction and compassion rather than the facts of the case. Any dissatisfaction must be at least in part due to some negligence on the doctor's end. The complaining party walks away with a pay day. And the attorney gets his/her cut of the winnings.

Embarrassingly, there is also that cadre of physicians who have been labeled "hired guns." They are frequently, though not always, respected members of the medical community who advertise themselves to med-mal lawyers. For a fee, they will manipulate a case history and find a tiny, albeit medically insignificant, break in the clinician's medical behavior—and, with a panache called "jury presence," will sway a relatively naïve panel and get a plaintiff decision. That fee is based on the potential payout and how creative they have to be. I have turned down many cases that in my opinion had not a shred of evidence of negligence; but, I would hear later through the med-mal grapevine that they found physicians who were given irresistible offers, and the cases had gone to trial.

Another fallout is that medical malpractice lawyers are sometimes publicly cast as the marquee villains in the litigious atmosphere that has run amok. One suggestion for control by the Bush II Administration has been to put a cap on awards with all sorts of formulas being suggested, none of which has been agreed to by any of the affected parties.

The Association of Trial Lawyers of America immediately got into it, fighting the administration all the way on this issue, what with those contingency fees based on awards. Loyal only to their own bottom line, they turned on the Democrats, as well, when the 2004 election slated a vice-presidential candidate who was a former med-mal attorney. He was GOP-marked and demonized à la Willy Horton as a "trial lawyer," almost as an epithet. The sobriquet stuck and did its job. Voter exit polls indicated that that demonization ploy proved to be quite successful.

The subterfuge used by oil companies and the utilities has been put into operation by the med-mal carriers. A threat of a huge increase in prices at the pump or at the electric meter is casually mentioned. Then, when a small portion of that request is granted by the state overseer agency or Big Oil, the unsuspecting buying public welcomes the "relief." This when the truth was that no increase at all was needed to maintain the services and their very ample profits.

That trick has caught on. The bugaboo of soaring malpractice insurance rates has been at the basis for many physicians crying poverty when they are faced with that reality. I do not recall a year when, as the July renewal rate for malpractice insurance policies loomed, that in early April, the insurance companies did not sneak in reports and comments in the lay press and medical journals that an increase in rates was applied for to the state insurance commission with great necessity in order to avoid a "crisis." Always with the adjoiner that bankruptcy was pending without it.

The facts always belied the truth. A recent Dartmouth College study showed again that falling or less-than-anticipated returns on investments by the med-mal carriers led to requests for increments in doctor/client premiums. Audits eventually consistently show that the malpractice carrier had always turned a handsome profit the year before. That insurance coffers were full to the brim and the payouts to attorneys and plaintiffs the year before came from interest on investments instead of actual premiums paid by doctors/clients. And remember, over 75 percent of courtroom decisions are in favor of the doctors/defendants. A smaller increase in rates is allowed, and the doctor community breathes a sigh of thankful relief as though they had won something.

Even President George W. Bush has insisted that payouts and frivolous lawsuits account for the raises in premiums. But this has been debunked over and over. Medical malpractice accounts for less than 2 percent of healthcare spending.

It seems that everyone is getting on the med-mal bandwagon. In a maneuver by the antichoice abortion movement in the Midwest several years ago (but apparently ongoing), a campaign got underway to conscript pregnancy termination post-ops who had had ever so slight "complications" from the procedure. They even used passing temperatures or mild discomforts that had been anticipated and were part of the patient consent and procedural information forms. Enough patients were found who had been naturally ambivalent and were in the throes of the dilemma over abortion. They were cajoled and enticed by the possibility of getting a sizeable cash payout (for them) when the doctor/abortionist would be sued for med-mal. Many bought into it.

The denouements were that since the cases were ill-based, just about all were eventually ruled frivolous by the courts and summarily dismissed in pretrial or never even got that far. I am not aware of a single case that went against the doctor or clinic. But they served a draconian purpose anyway.

Many clinicians were sufficiently annoyed by the hassle of the subpoenas and depositions, as well as the time and money spent to mount a defense, that they found it more practical to get out of the abortion business. That had been the only aim and expectation of the antichoice group in the first place. The medical malpractice litigious atmosphere was used in this special circuitous way. Mission accomplished.

In the past decade, the huge number of insurance claims has been flat. Only about 10 percent of those who have experienced any form of unexpected suffering following a medical intervention have ever filed a suit. A tiny fraction of doctors, just over 5 percent, accounts for over half of the malpractice payouts, the bad apple in the barrel theory. And state agencies have been generally reluctant to punish those doctors who are chronic abusers of the system. Just as in any private insurance company, the final premium rates are determined out of the experience of the whole. The good guys pay for the baddies.

So, what do we know now? That this crisis we hear so much about in the medical community is directly attributed to a for-profit healthcare system. The insurance company lobby well knows the meaning of a federal, national health system, when medical malpractice will essentially become a non-issue.

The Patient Bill of Rights

Yet another ploy used by the medical power structure has been to concoct other means that are seemingly on the patients' behalf. Posted in just about every doctor's office and certainly on every hospital and healthcare center bulletin board is the Patient's Bill of Rights (PBOR), usually printed on parchment-appearing paper, meant to resemble a page out of our Constitution.

This futile gesture, the PBOR, is just that—futile. Its intent is to give patients something in hand while picking their pockets. This is a form of incrementalism, a term FDR used back in the 1930s when he was exhorting Secretary Perkins to hold off against tacking a healthcare proviso onto Social Security for fear of losing both.

Just get your foot in the door, and we can open it wider and wider.

The Patient's Bill of Rights is one of those ruses. Dr. Marcia Angell, physician, activist/author, and former editor of the prestigious *New England Journal of Medicine*, has stated that, "Although we can all agree in spirit with the PBOR, they will not achieve their advertised ends. Rather, I am afraid, they will have effects opposite from those intended." Dr. Angell's reasoning, sadly, makes sense.

As employers continually fight against healthcare packages for their job force and attempt to do the bare minimum, the added costs attached to enforcing the Bill of Rights will have to be passed on to the employee. Who else? The more strict the regulations, the more the employers will opt out of the system, or what amounts to the same thing—make it so expensive the working group cannot afford membership.

The upshot of all this is that the Patient's Bill of Rights is yet another way of bamboozling patients into thinking a healthcare system based on privatization, "managed care," and profits is delivering the only thing needed—healthcare. Patients certainly do not want to be known as "clients." Hopefully, this will start to change as the sides are redrawn.

There is no doubt that rights—patients' and doctors'—are essential to any system. But you are putting the proverbial oil in water. Putting an alleged Bill of Rights in the middle of an already bankrupt system that does not deliver healthcare (read: the product) for all only distorts the whole gestalt further. Just as bosses are not good proxies for their workers, managed care is not a sound representation for the doctors. It is a non sequitur to suggest that these opposing forces are on the same side.

In "The Petition," a two-actor Broadway show performed in the mid 1980s by the real life husband and wife team of Hume Cronyn and Jessica Tandy, the plot centers about a London couple celebrating their fiftieth wedding anniversary, all done up in the elegant style of this legendary acting team. During their trips down memory lane through their marriage, Tandy confesses that she had a one-night sexual encounter in the seventh year of their marriage with no one other than their ceremony's best man, Cronyn's best friend.

"If it makes you feel any better," she commented, "he was always a gentleman."

Cronyn looks up with a half smile to his lips and remarks, "How could he have been a gentleman when he was in a place where a gentleman would never be?" ♦

The power mongers continue to conjure up various subterfuges and nuances that seemingly improve the system and correct its failings. But they are all cosmetics and more Titanic deck-chair shifting and nothing more. None end up with providing for those without.

More Smoke and Mirrors

That is where those two acronym agencies, HIPAA and COBRA, come into play. They are both directly tied into the Patient Bill of Rights phenomenon. They are both being presented now to patients as programs that are protecting those rights. It is not a tough sell but neither is it that clear cut.

The Health Insurance Portability and Accountability Act of 1996 authorized the Department of Health and Human Services (DHHS) to oversee and administer patient privacy. It was as though Congress realized the dearth of adequate healthcare in the nation and was doing what it could to cover it up by restraining communication. If no one talks about it, maybe no one will notice.

But how far does privacy go? We are not exactly sure what constitutes a break in those rules and regulations. For example, can nursing stations in hospitals continue to use slate boards that list room numbers and patient names and their attending doctors? Care has been taken to omit diagnoses and procedures from the board for all the public to see.

Certainly in the waiting rooms of public hospitals and clinics and very often in the private clinician's office, the next patient is called for his or her turn by name. Is that an invasion of privacy? Many a HIPAA authority has said yes. Or even the use of waiting room sign-in sheets, a frequent practice. Perhaps the solution is for the patient to take a number and be "next" like at the deli counter.

Caution must be taken by a doctor's office in using a patient electronic answering system to leave a message that just might be picked up by someone other than the patient. Or calls to a patient's home that results in a message of a medical nature left with a person, even if it is a spouse, sibling, parent, or significant other. No one is quite sure of what to do with the posting of patient names on hospital room doors.

The most disturbing enforcement of the HIPAA regulations came about when the doctors became confused as to how much information they could pass among themselves about patient care and conditions. The paranoia humor flows fast and furiously at many a staff meeting. A doctor is given certain privileged information very meaningful to a patient's medical condition—or perhaps peripheral, which happens often. The transfer of such information to a colleague comes under question. Doctors find themselves cutting a patient history short at a crucial moment, not knowing if it is permissible to go on. The doctor's smile is one of puzzlement.

HIPAA offers couched guidance. Hearing the subjective terminology of "careful" and "conscientious" and "reasonable," doctors often leave a HIPAA orientation session scratching their heads, wondering why they are suddenly being instructed, under potential penalties, to do what they always knew to be right, and essentially always did. Remember Hippocrates?

The American healthcare system, a result of a bevy of private enterprises run for profit and each with its own vested interest, is steeped with innuendos and arcane purposes of which HIPAA is only one example. It seems as though this obfuscation was done on purpose.

HIPAA was an inspiration that followed the federal and state governments' involvement in other industry controls, often after tragedies exposed the need. The 1984 holocaust at the Union Carbide pesticide manufacturing plant in Bhopal, India, that left 2,000 dead and more than 100,000 injured, somehow prompted Congress to act. The ins and outs of deciding who was responsible in Bhopal and at whose expense opened up the privacy issues on the whole. This led to the nation's first electronic disclosure requirement. Manufacturers were then forced to report annual release levels of toxic chemicals, facility by facility and chemical by chemical.

So-called chemical shaming led to other forms of regulations and disclosures. Dow, 3M, and Monsanto are among many other mega-manufacturers that were thus humiliated into self restraint, after studies showed that their manufacturing divisions were spewing millions of pounds of toxins into the world's atmosphere. When healthcare took its place as another privatized industry, it only followed that disclosure standards would eventually be put into place.

There is that other side of the coin. There are many healthcare authorities and think tanks that have expressed concerns over potential invasions of privacy that were once behind the HIPAA installation.

The original DHHS authorization law ordered Congress to act by August 1999. When that deadline came and went, President Clinton, in October 1999, proposed new regulations. They were not finalized until late 2000. Those revisions affirmed the legality of the HMO practices of perusing patients' records without patient consent. That is exactly what happened to my Jessica Riggins chart that made me so aware of such carryings on.

As Boston University School of Public Health Chairman George Annas said, "Everyone can see your medical record but you." Those rules do prohibit the disclosure of the medical records for marketing purposes or for employee hiring and promotion decisions. All of this is what is behind the entire HIPAA practice. Putting it into the context of the HMO system, it is essential to keep just anyone from finger-walking through patient files. Enforcing HIPAA challenges the whole HMO concept and its demands for full access to patient records.

Medical investigative reporter Kip Sullivan codified a long list of vague HMO-invented euphemisms that justify their intervention and allow their agents, as they did with Jessica Riggins, to get her vital signs and blood count before the floor nurses had them. These niceties include "conducting quality assessment and improvement activities" and "utilization reviews." Also "coordinating health plan performance" and Sullivan's acclaimed favorite, "management functions of a health-care provider or health plan." Now we know what they were doing when they were scanning Jessica's chart.

America is being inundated by the HMO insurance behemoth. Little by little, inch by inch, America's medical machineries are being swallowed up into the system. As patients start to realize their misgivings and become more disillusioned with the system, the HMO PR force swings into action. HIPAA is one of those little legerdemain tricks that keeps the patients/clients happy. It gives the impression that managed care is working for the public. Hence, all those euphemisms. More abound.

The accountability practice is being sold to the clients as for their own good and interests. Remember, with the new sides drawn up, pitting doctors and patients against HMOs and hospitals, the HMO takes on the role as the patient protector and often has to paint a shady picture of the doctor. Another use of demonization. Those "utilization review" and "quality assessment" euphemisms that were applied during my battle with the insurance people for Jessica Riggins were a way to soften the blow that the next step would be the "carve out" if I didn't comply.

HIPAA semantics do not leave anything to chance or, hopefully, future litigation risk. That is exactly what happened to Jessica Riggins. The HMOs have a free pass into patients' charts. The managed care people insist that this is all for patients' good, eliminating profligate hospital stays and exorbitant laboratory tests that will filter down to less costly care.

But in a managed care for-profit healthcare system, nothing of the kind happens. If it does, it is pure serendipity. Those corporate ethics and goals get in the way. First things first—a better end-of-year profit and loss statement for the company.

Snake in the Grass

COBRA, as noted, has an apt acronym. The 1986 legislation was ballyhooed as a guarantee that laid-off workers, whose jobs had included a healthcare perk, must be offered by their former employer the opportunity to purchase and maintain their existing coverage for up to eighteen months and at least at the same rate. This came out of the massive layoffs from the 1980 recession. The assumption is that the rates charged for the large employed group were more economical for the consumer than individual private insurers, something not always true.

This was about six years before President Clinton's spouse envoy met with that group at Jackson Hole and solidified the HMO ways and means. But the alleged benefits of COBRA were at the forefront of their HMO sales pitch and were used as part of patting their own backs for supposedly finally giving the country a bona fide healthcare package. COBRA was just one of the myriad of sleights of hand. Whatever very short-term benefits came out of COBRA, they quickly faded into oblivion. It is certainly now essentially a near useless program.

In opposing a national healthcare service, Hillary and her crowd insisted that COBRA was part of the answer as to how, while working within the system, they could take care of those in need. After all, the numbers make arithmetic sense. Those dismissed workers would have swelled the numbers of the uninsured even further and with great embarrassment. Now many of them would be "covered."

Think again.

There was even a fudging of the statistics. The ex-workers who were eligible for COBRA but who no how could afford such a benefit were counted in the group that suddenly had such coverage. This is like Washington's including the armed forces as among the working people so as to diminish the reported rates of unemployment.

What good is an available program when it is unaffordable? The government admittedly feared that the COBRA-provided people would have to scrounge for other coverage when the layoff goes past eighteen months, which is often the case. After the Reagan Medicaid slashes of the 1980s, those folks who lost their coverage but had managed to somehow accumulate some assets might not qualify for Medicaid, but in no way could come up with the price of a COBRA policy. That only exposed another cruelty in the system.

Many a scrounger discovered after a year and a half that the monthly cost of about $500 for a single person and as high as $1,200 for a family could easily be bettered if you did a little research and insurance shopping. People then also realized that for all the time on the job when there had been a healthcare perk, the plan chosen by management was not always the most sound, either economically or for the range of coverage. The plan was sometimes chosen because of the hard sell by the HMO sales force or payola at the top.

The *New York Times Magazine* recently ran a cover story about an unemployed computer worker who had been making almost six figures a year. His unpredicted and quite sudden layoff came when his wife was in the middle of her very expensive breast cancer chemotherapy treatments. COBRA came to cover $800 monthly, and the family assets did not qualify them for Medicaid. The food bill and the rent took priority, and so the chemotherapy was curtailed. They just crossed their fingers that enough had been taken. Stay tuned.

With such stories becoming commonplace in the work scene, and with audiences at political rallies becoming its victims, many pols who had previously hailed COBRA as a "Godsend" changed their tunes. And this happened in the *NYT* article to someone who was taking home three times the national average. The embarrassment comes about when there is no answer to audience queries as to what to do next. The answer usually is, "Punt."

It Can Get Worse

Some special groups are feeling the pinch of having no healthcare coverage more than others because their situations are relatively more severe. Paul Ginsberg of the Center for Studying Health Systems Change (HSC) put it this way. "Almost 5 million Americans face a triple threat. They have low incomes, they have ongoing health problems, and they have no health insurance." The present proposals in Congress that are going to be facing tough passage struggles these next few years do not address this issue.

Of those more than 45 million Americans that lack any form of protection, over 7 million suffer from chronic illnesses, which means their treatment patterns will likely go on for the rest of their lives. Many of those families of four fall outside the U.S. poverty scale that has been set at $35,000 annually. They become ineligible for any forms of coverage.

Just about every healthcare research organization looks at diabetes as a case in point. Its neglect has been pointed out as a glaring example of our lack of a national health system. Diabetes mellitus, the well-recognized condition caused by pancreatic failure to produce the hormone insulin that regulates sugar metabolism in the body, is a treatable chronic illness. And those that are treated lead relatively normal lives. But, if those over 15 million patients do not get regular doctor check-ups that ward off potential complications, very toxic side effects occur, such as blindness and amputation of affected limbs. It is therefore no wonder that statistics easily show that the uninsured and poorly insured have an outrageously many-fold increase in those very serious repercussions.

Other chronic diseases, which should get regular and constant attention but do not because of a lack of insurance coverage, affect millions of Americans, much more so as they get older. These tend to turn into those "pre-existing conditions" that are then denied by many carriers. Arthritis, clinical depression, asthma, and hypertension are some of those ailments with incidents measured in the tens of millions that demonstrate an age but not necessarily gender preference. There are also others that lead to high morbidity and mortality, are socially disdained, and are much more prevalent among inner city poor. They get dismissed and go underreported, like HIV/AIDS, hepatitis, and some forms of cancer.

The Bush II Administration and its cohorts up on the Hill deprive more and more Americans in so many fallout ways, such as tax credits for those in need and subsidies for employers. Those affected millions have no employers and are not employees. Their income taxes are a rate that any fanciful credit would be negligible. The most vulnerable are the first to suffer of being among the uninsured.

Prevention Instead of Cure

Ignoring the chronically ill—knowing that it often leads to preventable acute exacerbations that frequently, out of desperation, end up in the nation's emergency rooms and needing emergent Medicaid coverage—is a more foolhardy approach than ever. Computations have been made and presented to Congress in exactly this way, that such ER care is not only inadequate medically, it is a far more expensive way to deal with such a problem. As I said, the money is there. Just take it from where it is going.

There is no debate that acute care is more costly than prevention and proper management of chronic illness. But prevention is not the method of profiteering by those corporate healthcare moguls now in charge of the nation's healthcare.

Yet another vicious maneuver of corporate healthcare interests is playing the old game of pitting one faction of your enemy against the other. Divide and conquer. For example, they frequently divide those in need by age. The junior citizens are told they cannot and should not be held responsible for the elderly any more than is already being done (Medicare). The seniors are reminded that with their fixed incomes, they should not be taking on the care of the younger, and when brochures and promo pieces are put on billboards and in the mail, the youth are always pictured as those who appear drug-ridden, idle, ill-mannered, and unkempt.

There is, as well, the stand off between the early and late retirees. Those over sixty-five obviously qualify for Medicare. But the early retirees, some of whom have taken up such an offering from their employers as means of attrition rather than outright layoffs, are usually in the fifty-five to sixty year range and do not yet qualify for Medicare. Their fixed incomes in no way provide for taking on either a COBRA policy or private insurance. They then fall into the category of the uninsured. Some have had to reject an early retirement offer only because of the fear they will be without any semblance of healthcare coverage.

A report by the Washington-based Employee Benefit Research Institute stated that for these most recent years, retirees younger than sixty-five dropped from 22 percent to 13 percent. The nation's medical practitioners are facing this daily, as long-standing patients are coming in with heavy hearts and troubled voices, almost embarrassingly forced to admit to their doctors they are moving into retirement and may sadly not be able to keep up with their bills. COBRA was not an option, already having been considered and dismissed because of its cost.

"I just didn't know what to do," claimed one long-time generalist from Minneapolis. "How am I to dismiss a patient after so many years of loyalty and service? I'd look like an ogre, basing that relationship only on money. And yet, how am I to pay my own bills? I almost do not know what to tell these people. I am stymied." ♦

Bankruptcy

Well, maybe doctors aren't filing Chapters 7 and 13 so quickly, unless they have a filled three-car garage, a thirty-foot sailboat, and should be considering joining Gambler's Anonymous. Their only financial woes seem to crop up when the malpractice suit occasionally goes for the plaintiff and the settlement is in excess of the insurance policy coverage. But with just about all states now having umbrella policies that go over the required standard malpractice coverage, and with just about all judges tailoring the jury decisions to meet the insurance limits, that doctor out-of-pocket payout is rare indeed. But patients are constantly paying, that's for sure.

Bankruptcies and chronic ailments and debilitating injuries go hand-in-hand. The patients with injuries that prevent them from taking any employment opportunities, facing years of needed care, confront the frustration of mounting debt. Bankruptcy seems the only way out.

Medical expenses now account for more than half of the personal bankruptcies filed in the country last year. Rising healthcare costs, people without any medical insurance, and even out-of-sight deductibles that cannot be met by the patients are driving more people into bankruptcy after a medical crisis. There is a direct relation between the number of Americans without coverage and the number of personal bankruptcies that are filed.

But the Bush II Administration started to close that door, as well. In late 2005, the banking lobbyists earned their keep, when stringent new bankruptcy statutes went into effect, essentially denying that last bit of relief to those in financial straits. Even those who have lost everything following a medical crisis.

And contrary to the myth, the average profile of the debtor is not someone who needs AA or GA or who ran up foolish and huge credit card debts. It is a forty-one-year-old woman with two children and some college education who even owns her own home. She put off doctors' visits, which led to a more severe condition that resulted in a need for more acute and expensive care. Over half of those average filers had long histories of not filling needed but uncovered prescriptions. The more medications ignored, the more they became needed. and the ailments worsened. *Catch-22.*

The number of Americans who filed for bankruptcy in every recent year was in the hundreds of thousands. And many of these had some form of medical health insurance. There were those who lost their jobs during the long-term ailments and the insurance went with them. Still others got into real trouble when there was no way to meet the co-payments or deductibles and more, when the medical services needed were not covered by their policies. COBRA was beyond their budget. Other gaps in coverage popped up when it was discovered that they were part of the fine print in the policy statement that was sold to the gullible buying public.

One bankruptcy court hearing in California heard this sad tale. "I was just stunned when I heard the news from my personnel office. I thought I was covered for everything I might need. I hung on for as long as I could and then was let go when I couldn't get back on my feet in time. Sure, I was experienced and young enough, so I landed another position and a good one, too. But then more reality set in. My new insurance guys wouldn't take on my medical needs because of what they said was a preexisting condition. I actually tried to get my doc to fudge the records a little to make it seem like it was a new problem. And he was really sympathetic. We talked about it man to man, and he tried to help. There was just no way he could fake the deal. I understood. He tried. He really did." ♦

Washington has shown itself to be insensitive to this burning issue. In 2005, after credit card company lobbying, Congress made it more difficult to get out of a rampant debt. Houses and property are lost and the debt albatross hangs over your head for what seems an eternity. Future earnings are forever subject to levy.

Dr. David Himmelstein, associate professor of medicine at Harvard Medical School and author of many studies on healthcare crises and finances, finally admitted, "...if you are sick enough long enough, you're in deep trouble in our society."

Physician Behavior

HMOs are continually policing their providers to see to it that they meet the standards of practice in their community. Conventional medical literature distributed free to all medical practitioners ostensibly publishes articles that teach the medical offices various ways to maximize their profiling to up the ante paid out by the carrier. That is exactly like the rash of media ads by U.S. tobacco companies that urge children not to smoke and by whiskey brewers that advise against drinking.

But in the end, these canned medical journal articles, written by HMO staffers and put out under doctor bylines, pollyannically advise the doctors. They are to review patient scheduling to get the most patient visits, to put formularies for allowed medications in each examining room to avoid getting that call from the pharmacy that disallows the medication and necessitates writing another prescription, to review claim forms so double filing is not needed and to make sure all the blanks are filled in so they don't get returned and rejected for such frivolous and avoidable gaps. In the grappling between carrier and doctor, it is almost amusing to be an outsider and watch how each side tries their fencing manipulations so as not to be outsmarted by the other.

A multispeciality group in Dallas hired a sharp office manager who bragged that by taking all that advice, and therefore being a good and obedient player, he was able to negotiate a slightly better HMO contract the next time around. The business of America is business.

An internist of many years from a San Diego suburb had a dilemma. She had a patient of long-standing who was showing clear signs of bipolar depression and was facing a family crisis. An acute but short hospitalization was needed to get the fellow over the hump, but his insurance coverage's fine print was not about to allow the admission. "I told my patient to subtly hint that suicide was in his thoughts. That story should do it. It was a dilemma because I did not want that to go on his permanent record. But at his age, with no schooling or job searching in his life anymore, I figured it was worth the annoyance. At least it was a shared decision." ♦

Throwaway journals that get out to every doctor's office monthly always include an article or editorial with advice as to how the doctor should be handling the HMO to get a "better deal." A part of any well-staffed office includes, along with the nurse, lab tech, and patient assistant, a well-trained billing manager to cover the loopholes in the manipulations of the CPT codes and in signing an HMO contract. That position can be worth its weight in gold, as they say.

The HMO billers got wise to that game from the onset. Delayed payments and rejections comprise over one-third of the claims filed in any busy office. The longer their bank accounts are filled, especially at the end of each month when interest rates are calculated and awarded, the better the HMO bottom line.

"It wouldn't be so bad if health plans just made mistakes and you could take care of them with a phone call or two," said an active orthopedic practitioner in California. "But my experience is that these people are playing you for a fool. I really try my best to be legit. But I really think I practice fraud every day of the week with every billing I file with the HMOs. It has become a casual routine by my staff to try and outwit them. I feel dirty much of the time." ♦

HMO Tricks of the Trade and Their Deep Pockets

There is a litany of highly questionable HMO tactics. Here are some of their dirty tricks.

Downcoding. Just as the doctor becomes creative in his coding indices, the HMO office goes the other way and downplays the number. And in the heat of the day, a downcoding is not always recognized and gets by the medical office. HMOs actually have a special part of their staff for that purpose—to screen all doctor office billings for opportunities to downcode. They count on most of the payees to just accept the lower reimbursement rather than go through the rigmarole of wading through the maze of computer-answered phone voices, trying to find a human to plead the case. The doctor's office just throws in the towel and accepts it as the lesser of two evils.

Prior contracts. On occasion, a medical unit has signed two contracts during protracted negotiations with an HMO, likely in a rush to get back to attending the crowded and antsy waiting room. That office can be assured that the computer will be programmed to pay out on the lesser of the two. There have been offices that have caught that error after years of filing. The average doctor's office just does not have the billing staff and machinery to go back that far and fight for restitution. Nor did the doctor have time to read the fine print.

Standard fees for unique services and contracts. After a hard-fought battle to get higher fees for services rendered, the office has to keep an even sharper lookout to see if the new deal is being respected. It often is not.

Guarding the cap. After the office has negotiated a cap and is assigned a number of patients in that catchment area, the HMO insurer will often try to start the cap fees only after the patients have been seen. That might be months after the deal has been signed, which is definitely not the spirit or word of the cap arrangement.

Silent PPOs. Here the office will receive a lower payment, the HMO claiming that this is based on a prior contract signed with another HMO unit. That deal never existed. Fees are held in escrow until the scrap is settled.

Buried notification. Notice of fee schedule changes are often sent to the doctor's office as a part of a small print notification that even gets past an astute billing manager. The modern age of computer technology is an answer to that by programming it to match an individual payment against every billing.

Prior overpayments and takebacks. This is when those health plans audit themselves any time they want. It could be an honest error on their part, or more often, a deliberate review of whatever service was provided. The HMO decides there was an overpayment. A refund is requested. The statute of limitations for a takeback is not all that constant. Public Law 4406D says that the carrier must scan the doctor's catchment population to determine if his/her fees were out of line. There are also the individual arrangements made with the HMO and the enrolling doctor as to how far back it will be permitted to go when that type of audit is being made. Anywhere from one to six years are fair game. Just recently, a Cleveland pediatrician received a letter from an HMO that a prior takeback review was getting underway. The doctor's office manager was so astounded that she began a personal crusade in their defense of this HMO absurdity. In her response, she mused that should this happen, for example, after any doctor's death, the estate would be charged for the difference. Then it would be up to a stranger or non-medical heir to decipher the issues and settle with the HMO. Guess who would win?

The HMOs never lose. Never.

Withholds. The fine print in many a contract often has the HMO withhold a certain percentage of the fee for an arbitrary time period, which is at least until the end of that fiscal year or longer. If the HMO then decides there was any overpayment or change in fee schedule in its favor, the kickback comes out of the withhold. Or future earnings. There are now some restrictions being written into the law that are curtailing the insurance people from this practice.

They have been told by the state insurance authorities that it is not permitted to deduct payment from other coded invoices or other sources even though it is from that same medical office. They must fight it out and insist on repayment directly in the form of a reimbursement.

The HMOs never seem to lose. Never.

Is it any wonder why and how the doctors, without being cynics, are on the defensive when it comes to who is an ally? The doctors didn't trust the HMO when they signed the contracts; didn't have time to decipher the pages and pages of conditions, disclaimers, and loopholes, always in favor of the HMO; and therefore feel no loyalty when it comes to truth telling. One older practitioner at a staff conference advised calling the lying "judicious." That just made it sound nicer and even justified.

And the doctors are up against an insurance empire with staffs and attorneys and paralegals and funds galore. And all geared for action.

The HMOs never lose. Never. Well, almost never.

Those same medical journal articles then describe "solutions" to these very real problems. Like for the doctor to personally do the "yelling," as though that is all he or she had to do. Or hire two billing managers. Or three. Threaten the HMO with a collection agency and attorney. Stay in touch with your state's insurance commissioner, something I resorted to in the Jessica Riggins saga.

The carriers are well aware of the rancorous relationship that many providers feel exist between the two. Part of the sales pitch by the HMO to the doctor/provider includes reassurances that this issue is being addressed and that they are "on the same team." Yeah, sure. Then comes that small print.

A Colorado gynecologist managed to get a letter to the editor published in his state medical society's newsletter alerting his colleagues that the HMOs were allowing treatments for osteoporosis only when the standard Bone Mass Density (BMD) index came back from the lab at less than the critical 2.5 units, despite the patient's clinical condition and acclaimed need for relief. HMO medical care by the numbers. Practicing medicine without a license. ♦

That judicious fibbing is not limited to individual practitioners. Medical news reports in the lay press and medical journals also distort the truth in favor of their vested interest—product sales. One astute investigative reporter reminded her readers that "junk science," a term used to put down any opposing research, can include "checkbook science," or research designed not to enhance medical knowledge but simply to sell a product.

A freelance writer was looking for her next gig. A friend in medical PR had a suggestion. The drug companies were paying her firm big bucks to put together articles "written" by doctors coming out in favor of their latest and greatest wares. The writer could not resist. She paid her rent, the journal met its deadline, the doctor got a byline, the drug company promoted its product. Everyone won. Except John Q. Public, that is, who got the wool pulled over his eyes. He ended up paying a bill he never knew he owed. Or where it came from. Or why. ♦

The wined and dined clinicians are ever aware that the seemingly pedigreed speaker of the evening at a medical get together is a well-paid spokesperson for the drug house, HMO, or medical equipment company. A "Harvard report" or a "British medical society paper" or a "government project" is bantered about and that allegedly lends credibility to the speaker. They are never substantiated or clarified, but alluded to, and seem to refute data that were negative about the drug or medical procedure. In a world where the business of medicine is business, all is fair in love and war.

Copays, the vigorish the patient/client pays to the doctor/provider at each visit, are yet another sore spot, a point of contention between the physician and the managed care manager. They are also another reason why the doctor resorts to "judicious" lying and other alerts against the HMO in this antagonistic relationship.

The sad denouement of all this is that the HMO system and the corporate invasion into U.S. healthcare are no better exposed than when seen through the eyes of individual doctors in their constant parley with their HMO "partners." Fraud is so pervasive in the healthcare industry it becomes evident at every level.

Take Richard Scrushy, former CEO of HealthSouth Corporation, in 2003 the largest HMO provider of outpatient surgery, diagnostic imaging, and rehabilitation services in the United States. It operated over 1,700 rehab centers here and in Australia, Puerto Rico, and Great Britain. Scrushy blatantly pocketed more than a quarter billion dollars at the height of the fraud with assets that included yachts, Rolls Royces, Renoirs, Picassos, and a vault full of diamonds and platinum.

HealthSouth's over $4 billion in revenue and over 50,000 employees plummeted to barely 1 percent of its value within a year. That Scrushy and his board are facing jail time and financial ruin is small potatoes in comparison to the pensions and life savings lost by the thousands of employees. What happened at Enron and WorldCom was carbon copied.

HealthSouth is just one of many examples of what healthcare has become in the United States of America. It points out, so clearly, how allowing healthcare delivery to become a for-profit industry has opened the door to a myriad of deceptions and treacherous manipulations.

The Tug of War Is On

The American medical community is naïve when stacked up against the business moguls who now run the U.S. healthcare system. We doctors are definitely overmatched.

The doctors do have a number of weapons in their fight with the HMOs; they just have to be willing to use them. That "judicious" lying can sometimes get a patient coverage that would otherwise have been denied. By that minor switch in the billing code that cannot be refuted, doctors can get more of what they need.

There is a dilemma here. Ethical physicians are disturbed by untruths, and patients, even those who could gain from the doctors' massaging the diagnostic codes, are often uneasy. They may feel that if the doctors will fib to an HMO, they will fib to them. Doctor John and his wife scared off my patient that way.

Trying to convince the public that the doctor is Robin Hood, the HMO is Prince John, and the hospital is Sherwood Forest is a tough sell. In a sense, the physicians have brought this cynical approach on themselves, but if only out of economic self-interest, they have been aroused. Maybe medical schools should add a business management course to their curriculum so that graduates will be prepared to face the rigors demanded of them by a modern medical practice.

An old English adage attributed to maybe Shakespeare or Samuel Johnson has it that one lies for two reasons. One is that the truth would be hurtful and/or damaging; the other is that you are reacting to and mimicking a liar.

Now that the sides have been drawn, it is becoming clear that the patients and the doctors must watch each other's backs and remain allies—as they have been through the ages. Until healthcare takes its rightful place in our social order, Hippocrates, wherever he is, will just have to don the blindfold of Justice.

CHAPTER 10

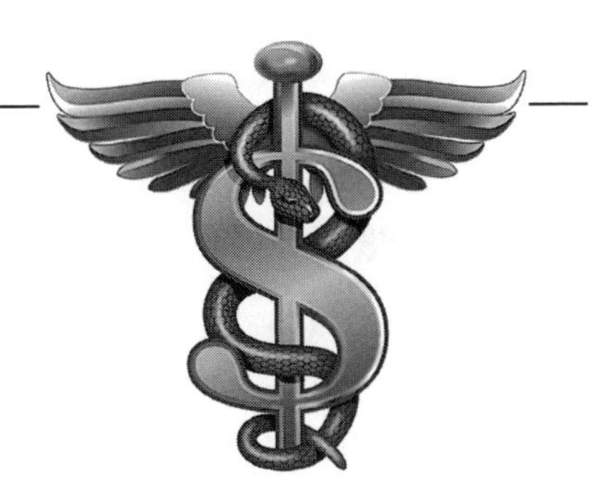

The Condition, The Situation, and the Cause

Aristotle wrote that there is a condition, a situation, and a cause to every event.

The condition here is a world that is bound and controlled by capital-based economies. Economies that profess that free enterprise and a floating market are the way to go, and put their faith for growth and development in hegemony, manifest destiny, and fee-for-service, with profit always the hallmark for accomplishment. Ronald Reagan called it "supply side economics." For George W., it's "ownership America." These men and their fiscal advisors always insisted that the amassed wealth by the haves would trickle to the have-nots. That theory just never seems to work out in practice.

The situation is that in this country, healthcare has been thrown into the economic pie, where its provisions follow the tenets and ethics of capitalism, and profits are still the criteria by which we mark success.

Then there is the cause—the doctors who, at the head of the pack of healthcare professionals, act as the key suppliers of such services. The doctors who, as Cuban Presidente Fidel Castro calls them, are shepherds, with the training, experience, and expertise to provide their flock with arguably their single-most essential need—health.

That significance cannot be exaggerated. Their import cannot be aggrandized. The meaning cannot be enlarged.

The healthcare industry is now the third largest in America, following the government and the whole of retailing. A recent Democratic Party white paper described the "30-30" problem, noting that 30 percent of our entire economy goes toward health and medical costs but adding, sadly, that 30 percent of our citizens have no regular contact with the medical system—the type of contact that is required for all of us to get the quality of healthcare that would be optimum and which America can well afford.

But in this healthcare industry of ours, it all boils down to that bottom line—profit and business success.

So let's put aside that given for the moment, that no work or play can even begin without good health, and talk about what is taught to every child in the country—the importance of money. Money, money, money. It's what makes the world go round, as the song goes.

I guess it is just not like I imagined. I grew up in a medical household. I am a third-generation doctor. My grandfather, Popop, used to take me with him every once in a while when I was a tot out on his house calls. He told me that although he was just starting out when The Depression was shaking off its doldrums, he went out and bought a new car that he could hardly afford because he felt that his patients would feel more confident if their doctor pulled up in a decent vehicle instead of a broken down jalopy. He had a spotlight installed at the driver's door that he adjusted from the inside so he could illuminate the house numbers and street signs. Especially helpful in his later years when his eyesight was not what it used to be.

Sometimes I would go into the patient's house and wait for Popop to finish. I would get a cookie for my troubles. I remember we would get back home and he would tell Momom that the patient was short that month and the only payment was the cookie.

Even my dad was somewhat traditional. Popop and Dad were both generalists and took care of all comers, from oldish kiddies to old folks. It kind of depended on their whims at the time. When it came to my turn, the house call was fading away and the fancy technology of modern medicine almost required the patient get to the office to get the best diagnostic workup and testing. Made sense.

But much more than that has changed. The medicine I recall from Popop and Dad just doesn't exist anymore. And worse, the relationships between doctor and patient have changed. Yeah, it would still be better to pull up in a spiffy car with a spotlight at the driver's door and have a state-of-the-art office to impress the patient. That assumes this translates to your ability as a physician. That is the thinking.

Nowadays, either with capitation or people just sent over from some HMO office, business is business. Everything is different. ♦

Perhaps it is just syllogistic. While we are pondering over and debating that conditional adjustment, we are faced with a situation that history and experience have shown us can be improved. The healthcare industry is just too important to leave up to amateurs and business people. This must all start with the acceptance that it is one "business" (along with education) that cannot put business ethics and motivations before quality of service.

To be even more practical, it is the physician community that must take the reins and fight for themselves and their patients. For it is they who have the education, articulation, and presence to make a change. There is no logical way we can expect the people to organize and demand the healthcare they are entitled to without their doctors at their side. This is the start of something big.

Who Will Pay?

If it is to be, it is up to me. ♦

Most in Congress say that universal healthcare is "impossible." That has been asserted by the Senate GOP majority leader, Tennessean Doctor Bill Frist, who, with his family, is an owner of that largest healthcare HMO/hospital combine in the country. The sadder part of it is that this is surely not true, even allowing for the profits built into our healthcare system. Take those away and we'd have a virtual bargain basement.

It gets worse. As the average costs go up, up, up, income goes down, down, down. The Kaiser Family Foundation and the Research Educational Trust (RET) have published their 2005 report that is considered a definitive measure of what coverage will be costing America's workers and their employers. It found that average annual premiums for family coverage grew 9.2 percent since 2004, to a whopping $10,880, more than the average worker in the same class had as an average minimum wage before take-home pay of $10,712! Some make more, many make less. Kaiser added that since 2000, healthcare premiums have gone up over 70 percent; wages have increased 15 percent.

Meaning? That job-based health insurance, the central linchpin of what the USA calls a healthcare system, and what Hillary Rodham Clinton and her Jackson Hole conclave gave the people a decade ago, is now bent to its breakpoint. The employers, as the rates climb, are phasing out healthcare as a job incentive, knowing their competition will not upstage them. The results? Those workers just go without. That is why the naked 45 million in the country will be measurably more by the time you wake up tomorrow morning.

If you think healthcare is expensive, try sickness. ♦

So let's talk about healthcare financing, and let's put those many myths aside once and for all.

If we again are reminded of Silent Cal's adage that the business of America is business, the evidence clearly shows that those developed Western countries with a semblance of national health services and a single-payer system are good for business. Business leaders themselves have always complained that while they are forced to admit the health services purchased are not quality as compared to those other nations, their biggest beef at the board meetings is that "we are paying too much." So why, oh why, does corporate America turn its back on a publicly financed system that the taxpayers would surely support if given the chance?

The answer is not going to satisfy all because it seems to be illogical. A further review of the statistics tells us where we are and what we need. A single-payer, publicly financed healthcare system would end up costing the employers less in taxes than they now spend for their private health insurance. The annual $40 billion workman's compensation would go into the healthcare pot; auto insurance rates would fall after eliminating that needed portion of the premium that accounts for accident coverage. There would be additional positive repercussions.

Corporate America not only refuses to support a national health service, it actively fights against it. We have seen that, following the most recent closest point we ever came to getting an NHS—at Jackson Hole, when the White House met with the moguls who govern the government. And they walked away without getting any closer.

In those years following Jackson Hole and the first Bush *fils* Administration, healthcare has shrunk in the country. The uncovered grow, Medicaid and Medicare get under funded, and the private carriers price themselves out of business and just continue to diminish services.

The prediction by government statisticians is that as we near 2010, healthcare will represent a total outlay from all sources in the USA at over $2.5 *trillion*. The filtering down goes deeper. In this very competitive world, with Asian industries and the various free-trade pacts opening up Third World working forces, U.S. workers are becoming more and more "unaffordable" as reported by a survey in the Kaiser Foundation of 3,000 U.S. companies.

The Foundation noted that between 2001 and 2004, there was a loss of nearly 5 million jobs in the U.S. only because of that unaffordability of healthcare coverage. On the presidential hustings of 2004, as the Bush/Kerry camps debated some healthcare issues, we learned that rising premiums lead to a deterioration of the quality of jobs, in that other perks were curtailed to meet the company budget. The overall job market was decidedly slower where the healthcare package was comparatively larger, but the other perks were curtailed. In the industries where the healthcare perk was smaller, those jobs held their own. Obviously because vacation schedules and other niceties were what attracted the potential employee.

Their extreme was even more alarming and glaring. At the top of the list was generalized manufacturing, where the benefits cost 18 percent and job losses were at the same 18 percent. But in the accommodation service industries, healthcare was only 12.5 percent of the perk package and jobs *grew* at over 2 percent. Quite a difference.

Many a strike and job action in these past five years has not been so much over wage increases, which, in fact, were expected and offered (even if only to match the cost of living indices), but a cessation of healthcare coverages. American working families are becoming more and more aware (read: scared) of what is happening to their healthcare plans and know they cannot do without. Not for one minute. They walk the picket lines more readily for that than any other reason.

More filtering down and more fuel for the fire. The industry CEOs are infighting, in that they are almost but not entirely unified on the issues. DaimlerChrysler has consistently broken ranks with the rest of its industry in calling for an NHS rather than maintain the status quo and keep their private insurance carriers.

That comes down to another quirk that is damaging to the struggle and creating a havoc of its own. As the U.S. becomes more and more two-job family units, strictly out of economic need and survival, one of the family workers will be in an industry that offers some sort of health package, while the other will often be in one either with miniscule coverage or with none at all.

Just take the nation's largest private employer, Wal-Mart. Their over 2 million employees are listed surreptitiously as part-time and get no benefits; the full-timers merely get the way to purchase a company-sponsored plan, an expense most cannot afford and therefore bypass. They go naked. There are other companies that have followed that example, especially in the fast food industry.

Now we are left with a family unit that has one of the working members "cover" the healthcare of the other worker in the family. For just one example, well over half of PepsiCo's employees are better covered by someone else's insurance. The employee with the superior family coverage is usually in an industry that is facing global competition, while the beneficiary, with lesser coverage, is in an industry that is essentially competition free.

That seeming unfairness has caused many a rift among the members of management and is another reason why they have not been unified. Those bankruptcies mentioned earlier are taking a toll on families. That may well be the most shameful and evident social economic indictment of how the U.S. treats its indigent sick. If this were back a couple of hundred years ago, the poor houses would be filled with those who were escaping debtor's prison for not being able to pay their doctors and hospitals.

Credit cards are among the ways many patients get into trouble. And it seems that it is almost a conspiracy. No matter what kind of financial difficulties you are trying to bail yourself out of, with a Chapter Thirteen at the top of the list, solicitations from credit card companies and banks are mass-mailed daily.

Many people have become desperate enough to sign on the dotted line of a credit card application received in the mail with penalties and interest rates on the unpaid debts that seem usury. Indeed, they are.

Over 3 billion such solicitations are sent out yearly, about a dozen for every American man, woman, and child. They then find themselves some temporary relief by using the card to pay off their medical bills, seemingly forgetting that the end of the month will eventually come around.

In 2001, the credit card companies brazenly lobbied Congress to tighten the bankruptcy laws, and it obliged in 2005, making it that much more difficult to file because of credit card encumbrances. And many of those victims of this system even have some form of health insurance. In one survey of bankruptcies following credit card debt, over three-quarters had had some form of health insurance at the start of the illness. That was still not enough to keep them out of harm's way. Chronic and long-standing illnesses in the family will lead eventually to job loss. There goes the coverage.

COBRA, as we now know it, is not the answer. Here comes Chapter Thirteen, if you can meet the new stringent requirements, that is.

We are all now aware that General Motors prefers to put together its product across the border in Canada rather than in Detroit, knowing they will not have to account for healthcare and thus save that $1,500 per assembled auto. This is repeated over and over in that industry and others that are getting the message.

It remains an enigma why DaimlerChrysler, for example, cannot sway Ford or GM to hop on the single-payer public bandwagon. Every healthcare endorser eventually admits that an NHS will not come to fruition until organized labor joins in the struggle.

An NHS program got a big boost just recently when the National Association of Manufacturers (the same NAM that was strongly behind Morris Fishbein and the AMA back in the 1930s in fighting off FDR and Frances Perkins from adding an NHS as a Social Security rider), the U.S. Chamber of Commerce, and even the omnipotent Business Roundtable (BRT), an association of over 150 mighty CEOs with nearly trillion dollar budgets, were reportedly at least considering not vocally opposing an NHS.

But somehow, that hasn't changed the general tempo. Big industry has not come aboard, despite what seem to be obvious advantages. Are they still living in the Morris Fishbein/Joe McCarthy era, when a fellow traveler is lurking around every corner and some sort of a Kremlin spy is behind any governmental intervention? Are they afraid that if the government takes over healthcare, they are next?

Could that be it?

We Are All Connected

Even if we had managed to pull off an honest election in 2000 and 2004 and Al Gore or John Kerry had prevailed, an NHS would have no way been automatic, despite what both said on the campaign trail. Remember that Bill Clinton gave us that same hogwash back in 1991 and we ended up with Jackson Hole and the HMOs. But it might have brought us a step closer.

The issue that has been bantered about is that since we have not been able to sell national healthcare as a moral issue and appeal to that sensitivity of those in charge, why not sneak in the back door and sell it as good business sense? After all, they are business people. Whatever, it has not yet seemed to work.

Because of the importance of the business community, the healthcare movement is continuing to aim their selling program at the NAM and the BRT. Makes more sense. Like I said, if you think healthcare is expensive, try sickness. When American working people get sick, the whole nation suffers. The toe bone and head bone are connected.

Absenteeism from the job costs all of us hundreds of millions of dollars annually, and most of that is attributed to preventable conditions. That includes workers who take sick days to care for themselves because they did not catch their conditions in time. Or they stay off the job to care for loved ones for the same reasons.

The report *Health and Productivity Among U.S. Workers* stated it clearly enough. "We've been talking too much about how it costs to provide health insurance and not enough about what we lose as a country and as employers by having employees who are too sick to work." The report also coined the term "presenteeism," being on the job but not being able to concentrate or perform optimally. That included the many millions who did not have the prescription drug coverage and then never took the simplest of medications that would have nipped the malady in the bud and gone a long way to prevent that wasteful absenteeism.

It is a two-edged sword. When the need to stay away exceeds those sick days allowed, which is often, the lost wages make it that much more difficult to get the needed meds the next time around. Catch-22.

The pace of healthcare spending seemed to have leveled off a tad in 2003 but then took off again in 2004. That is the year it topped 15 percent of the GDP. There is a cruel codicil to that, as well. We continually get reports and memos issued by the federal government that seemingly boast of our curbed spending or brag how we held the line on payments to nursing homes, hospitals, and clinics. But those issued statements never add the draconian data that tell of closed medical centers, curtailment of medical staffs, and shortages in equipment and meds.

Medical ethicists (whatever they are) are looking at how the added costs of coverage to either Medicare or the privates affect patient care. Patients become the decision makers as to how and when they will seek medical care. This is not always based on their aches and pains, but solely on their ability to pay the piper.

Over the years, I learned that many a patient did not fill my prescription due to lack of coverage. This is becoming more and more commonplace as drug coverage allowances become more confusing and deficient. I would later discover that they did not return to me or their other doctors out of that same concern. As I said, that is the only time I have ever scolded a patient.

I get my dander up when I am told by a patient that he or she didn't want to bother me at an off hour. Then I remind them who and what I am and why I pay a telephone answering service a bunch of money every month for just that purpose—so patients can reach me on off hours.

Then I get more of the truth. That they didn't have the money in hand to come in for another visit. I feel like screaming but I keep my cool and remind the patient, although in a stern tone, that the only way to annoy me and make me angry is not to call when needed. I often try to add some subtle humor by chiding the patient for not liking me. When I get an expected quick denial, I ask them if they like me so, why not make my life easier by calling me at once and we get in the quick fix instead of letting the condition get out of hand. They get the point. It doesn't happen again. ♦

I am well aware of the bad apple in the barrel theory. We tragically have those practitioners who have become so cynical by the system that they treat patients based on capitation or whether they have the insurance or deep pockets to back up their calls for help. Shame on the doctors for that. They are the ones who should stand up in front of a mirror, in their birthday suits, raise their right hands and take the Hippocratic Oath all over again. *Primum non nocere.*

Of the nearly 125 million ER visits yearly in the U.S., a little over three-quarters are referred on to private office care. A study was done by the AMA to see what happens to patients who are seen for what they deem are emergent concerns but, after "appropriate management and control," are referred on to private doctors' offices for follow up. A set of research assistants posed as patients and went through that callisthenic.

The results were a sad, sad commentary on the U.S. medical community. Unfortunately, the type of coverage had something to do with what happened next. Those who claimed they had private insurance were decidedly able to see their private doctors sooner than those with Medicaid. Each "patient" in the study made several calls to different offices, generally related to their staged concerns. Just about all specialists were included in the group.

The report noted that the callers to just about all the offices were rigorously screened for their coverage, and most even received a return call to verify residence and insurance policy info. Privately insured patients were seen twice as fast as the Medicaids. When the "patients" said they would be able to pay a part of the requested fee or when they said they would pay in cash in full, there was little difference in the timing of the appointment. I guess the office manager just figured that showing such good faith as having some up-front money was at least a start.

What should patients do who are either on Medicaid or have no coverage at all and are in desperate need of help? The tongue-in-cheek advice is to either tell a judicious fib to get coverage or just not get sick.

Primum non nocere.

Yet another way the HMO insurance carriers have found to limit what they consider excessive use of the services is to simply increase those co-pays and deductibles. Insurance company spokespersons are always clamoring over "pampered patients" who "abuse" the system. One of the biggest selling points to personnel departments at management is to talk about small deductibles, which then become selling points to the workers, who then are reminded that their bosses have negotiated "the best deal."

Deductibles and Other Shenanigans

But with the encouragement of the AMA, the GOP Administration, and the American Hospital Association, among others, larger deductibles are on the top of every agenda when it comes to crunch time at the HMO.

It is all part of the "blame the victim" game. When the deductibles are increased, the company comes back with the excuse that something has to be done to stop the abuse of services, and so higher deductibles will weed out the abusers and make it better for everyone. The subterfuge also includes terminology to fit the crime. They are not called higher deductibles by the HMO; the term applied is "defined contribution plan." That is like Bill Frist claiming that when HCFA allows more for HMO Medicare fees it will create more competition and drive down prices.

Managed care thinking also teaches the workers that by having a higher deductible and that allegedly lower premium, they are getting more involved in the process and will therefore be more alert to higher doctor fees and hospital costs and can then protest. Patients are thus being turned into healthcare consumers.

The reality? That with this manipulative, fee-for-service additive, patients will naturally tend to put a dollar in their healthcare perspectives and will suffer because many will be forced to opt to avoid needed care, rather than look with dread to that big pinch at the end of the month when the rent, telephone, and electric bills come due.

An incentive is also part of this scheme. To get the higher deductible accepted and "bought," the HMO then cuts a little off the price of the total policy. But when you do the math, the costs of the deductible always exceed the policy decrease.

HMOs, like their insurance company parents, never lose.

The high costs that are hidden with all the sleights of hand by the HMO are easy to pick out and identify. They include, in no order of size or importance, those high administrative costs that are in excess of every other NHS in the developed world, sometimes double; higher fees claimed by doctors when they learn to manipulate the system in their favor; grotesque prices charged by the pharmaceuticals; and, of course, the offensive million dollar salaries tendered HMO CEOs or hospital administrators who play ball, plus their similar benefits packages, those golden parachutes and retirement pensions, well into the millions annually and the profits tacked on to placate the stockholders.

A million here. A million there. As they say, before you know it, you are talking real money. It all adds up. That is what we are getting for our fee-for-service medicine we are living with in the USA.

Want yet another *non sequitur*? There have been analyses bought and paid for by the HMO people to show that with those higher deductibles, healthcare final bottom line costs decrease. Yes, those numbers are valid. But beware. The kicker is that they are lower because there is lower healthcare utilization.

The consumers polled admitted avoiding that year's PAP smear or that very much needed hypertension follow-up office visit. That a medical need decision was a burden on the consumer/patient tells us the expected—that patients are not able to properly tell the differences between the necessary and unnecessary when it comes to their own health needs. It is like that saying "a physician who treats him/herself is treated by a fool."

As that high-deductible trick is coming more and more into vogue, it is being adopted by the managed care prescription drug benefits plans. With higher copays and deductibles attached to prescription drug plans, study after study has shown that the higher the copay, the more often the needy patients duck out on renewing the drugs at times when they cannot come up with the copay tariff.

Slot machines! I can see it all now: I need an appendectomy. Let's go pull on the one-armed bandit or bet a few bucks on 34 red and the pass line to raise the dough.

Gimme a break!

That incrementalism has been a ploy by many a political/activist group, and it has proven to be valuable in many campaigns. The theory to "get your foot in the door" has been successfully used time and time again. That is why opponents of any action seem to carry on in excess to prevent the smallest compromises in the big picture. Once the crack has occurred in the dike, the wall often comes tumbling down. But as already said, incrementalism has no place in the struggle for healthcare in America. It is too unique an issue.

In fact, local-type healthcare plans are formulas for failure. And while they are experimented with as possible solutions, valuable time is lost and funds and energies are wasted. The only real value to the states clamoring over providing healthcare for its people is to remind the nation as a whole and the federal leadership that there is no more pressing a need. Hopefully, it will serve as a wake-up call to every administration in Washington to get started down that road. The squeaking joint will one day get the oil. We just need more squeaks.

There are conflicts of interest popping up all over the place. If and when locals announce some sort of plan to implement a healthcare system, the feds do what might be expected. They add a new justification to their lack of attention and funding by merely stating that since the state and major cities are putting a program together, the federal agencies need not bother.

The conclusion from all these noble efforts (more smoke than fire) is that there is no place for individual local programs in the struggle to achieve a national health service.

Period. End of story.

No state has the wherewithal to either orchestrate or maintain such a program, much less the personnel at any administrative level to even blueprint such a thing. I've said that before; I will say it again and again. Only the federal government in Washington has that scope, ability, personnel, and funding.

National problems demand national solutions.

Canada and Great Britain Revisited

The demonization of the Canadian and British healthcare systems has taken on an entirely different facies. Now that there are no "Roosians" and their Kremlin to jump on, "socialized medicine" and its implications have been transplanted. Similar message. Same purpose. Just a different set of players.

Since the comparison is always made between ours and the other G-7 countries with their forms of healthcare, aimed mostly at the doctor community, the HMO propaganda mills and PR people are always quick to report any signs of failings in the Canadian, British, French, and Australian healthcare systems. And it seems that just as physicians swallowed the AMA bait back in the 1930s, they are taking big gulps out of the present hullabaloo over foreign healthcare programs.

No question about it. The British NHS is in trouble, even though it still is the only medical access for about 90 percent of the British people. A survey of London and five other major English cities showed that medical equipment there is becoming outdated and outmoded with replacements and upgrades coming not nearly quickly enough.

The Tory group, with ex-PM Margaret Thatcher having paved the way, granted favor to the Private Financing Initiative (PFI) with an attempt to shift budgets away from the NHS. On the other hand, happily so, there is also a bitter fight brewing against any leaning toward privatization. Hospital strikes and protest walkouts have been staged as the battle heats up.

The British media themselves have frequent, near daily articles and programs describing the long waiting times for operations, as well as nursing shortages and lengthy outpatient clinic queues. These are all above and beyond what would be expected and acceptable in such a vast and complex delivery system.

But it is the loudest secret ever kept that the U.S. and British media are joined at the hip. The Rupert Murdoch media empire is not the only one, by far. They both have the same vested interests. The same advertising clients. The same interlocking directorates.

That goes the same for the electronic media. That *New York Times* silence (I guess it was not news fit to print) is not the only one that brought the rank and file to protest. The four major American TV networks are wholly owned and operated by major U.S. corporate interests, namely General Electric, Westinghouse, Disney, and Murdoch News Corporation. Their links on all levels with the insurance conglomerates give the managed care private health industry quite an edge in getting out their message to the people.

But although no system has been more vilified by its detractors, NHS supporters are holding the line. The UK system is among the closest example the capital world has come to socialized medicine. Not only are physicians salaried, making it come that close to a true national health service, Parliament has also, as a part of the statutes, negotiated with domestic and international drug firms in order to keep prescription medication prices within reason, something that is glaringly disallowed by the 2005 Medicare rule preventing the HCFA from doing the same.

Two boasts have always been heard by the NHS supporters—and they have stood the test of time. One is that 100 percent of Brits receive healthcare, and two, that it is essentially very cost effective.

There have been many person-on-the-street interviews on both sides of the Atlantic on the healthcare issue. A wide range of American adults, even those with a modicum of coverage, have clearly expressed a certain uneasiness and anxiety. There is little trust that Washington will not further erode their present plan and also the apprehension that in the face of a job layoff, they will be unable to protect themselves and their families with a COBRA policy.

But their counterpart street Brits, despite their concerns for waiting periods and services and other perceived shortcomings, preface their remarks with a sense of security that is not seen in the USA. They express a basic comfort, knowing that at least during their most difficult times, they will have basic medical care.

The prestigious Commonwealth Fund completed a massive study two years ago that compared just about all aspects of the American, English, Canadian, New Zealander, and Australian systems. Its conclusion was an embarrassment for the United States. Despite all their deficits, the complaining from men and women in the streets was loudest when Americans had to face the HMO managed care thrust at them and live with a fee-for-service system.

What is the fodder for the cannons of the HMO propaganda machine? The answer is simple and evident for all to see. That the Thatcher policies, still being followed by the Labour PM Tony Blair, were continuously and are currently cutting funding from the NHS. That bottom line is their bottom line. Every budget over the Blair years has seen drops in support for the NHS. So it is no wonder that there is grumbling within the ranks of the salaried doctors and other healthcare professionals.

The John Conyers HR 676 and the Barbara Lee HR 3000 have borrowed many pages from the English NHS, just as so many others have from the best of the U.S. Constitution. Both, therefore, would be a start in the right direction.

Closer to home, and pictured as just as big a demon, is the Canadian healthcare system. That system is also, it seems, always fighting off the privateers. In the mid-1960s, the Royal Commission of Health Services was established, which Canadians refer to as Public Medicare. The 1984 Canadian Health Act defined and reaffirmed for the first time the basic adages needed to spell out healthcare provisos. They included covering all maladies and patient ailments, having it available to all its citizens, no exceptions, and that it be standard throughout all the provinces that they pay their set share of the coverages—but that it was set up to have guaranteed financing, no matter who does the paying.

Yes, there have been constant bombardments by the private sector that have, like Mother England, stripped the healthcare budget to a point of sometimes crying "Ouch!"

The Canadian system has revealed two glaring advantages over its stateside neighbor to the south. That the costs per citizen year after year are less than half of the U.S., and that bureaucratic expenses are also half of its American counterpart with its privatization.

The political scuttlebutt on the streets has it that no government, Labour or Tory, would ever tamper with the basic Canadian system, admitting it would be political suicide at the next election.

Finally, the French healthcare system, not literally a national health service run by the federal government, uses a different machinery to accomplish the same ends. Although the system may not be applicable to a vast cosmopolitan country more than four times France's size and scope, the USA could borrow valuable lessons in cooperation.

Ranked overall number one in cost effectiveness by the World Health Organization (WHO), the French program is truly universal and jointly controlled by labor and employers' organizations. Contrary to the U.S., labor is not seen as a special interest in France. Through its *Mutuelle Funds,* the French labor unions have joined up with other branches of society to combine their efforts to see that all its citizens are covered. None of them have adopted positions of antagonism or opposition nor do they feel threatened by the others.

France's healthcare system is actually a working combination of the public and private sectors. It was formed in the harsh years of Nazi occupation that politically tore the country apart and the immediate aftermath of World War II. France was rocked by sectors of the government that yielded obsequiously to their German occupiers and were later tried and punished severely as collaborators.

Post-war French psychology called for a marked rebound unity and peace among themselves. The *Mutuelles* with their remarkable labor-management cooperation have gained enormous respect by political observers worldwide.

In the U.S., General Motors, for one example, has expressed envy over that cooperation that is not seen in the States and is eyeing the Canadian system across their border from Michigan and those potential savings at the manufacturing level borrowed from their Franco counterparts. There is that ever prevalent sense that U.S. labor unions, fearful of losing their bargaining chip to attract new members in offering healthcare coverage they do not have otherwise, shy away from throwing their weight into the battle for a true national healthcare service here in the U.S.

The French *Mutuelles* have no such fear. With a "Medicare" program also in effect, and with virtually everyone (99.9 percent), employed or not, covered by public health insurance, France is closest to being the world's only industrialized nation with true universal coverage and with true total access to its entire healthcare system.

There are gaps, as expected, with the as-yet fragments of private care. There are small but ever present out-of-pocket payments by the patient, and dental and vision care expenses are largely not yet included. Those are on the French drawing board for the years to come.

Yet another way of undermining the movement for a national health service is by spreading the thinking that we don't have too little healthcare, we have too much! And that by just cutting down on the excess would save enough to cover those who now go uninsured.

President George W. Bush does not seem to ever miss an opportunity to foolishly claim that we have the best healthcare in the world. As always, he speaks for the haves, not the have nots. The U.S. system has left us with those who have all they need and then some in every economic aspect of life, and the many without enough or any. I wonder what Joe McCarthy and Morris Fishbein would have to say about that. "The Roosians are comin'!"

Talk show host Bill Maher noted late one evening that the medical community is still using maggots and blood-sucking leeches for various accepted medical indications. He then added that he thought we already had been using those things for various maladies all along, only we call them HMOs. ♦

Race and Gender

Since the healthcare issue is but a microcosm of the nation as a whole, it is no surprise that racism and sexism have played their parts. As the number of those without coverage increases, the number of women and those of color who suffer enlarges disproportionately. Many surveys have shown that the financial burdens of private health coverage are more of a sting on women and African-Americans and other people of color.

Several state-wide surveys have shown that young adults and blacks are more likely than the general population to be without health insurance, and three-fifths of the working insured are employed in the service sector that have scant health perks. Remember, the country's largest private employer, Wal-Mart, has essentially no coverage for its work force. That task often falls onto an already burgeoning Medicaid system.

We have thankfully come a long way since the Reconstruction Period, the Ku Klux Klan, and the rampant segregation of the earlier part of the twentieth century. Along with marked public washrooms and drinking fountains for "coloreds," there were actually separate hospitals. All Southern cities, even some in the North, came to know which were "Black" hospitals and which were "White."

World War II's awareness of the rabid Nazi racist policies, the Civil Rights movement, the expansion of health programs (i.e., Medicaid and Medicare), and the social impact of the Vietnam decade made Americans more cognizant of people of color worldwide and our racist crimes at home. These were the principle factors that opened up medical and nursing schools to all comers. However, the residue of racism is still very much alive. Neighborhoods still reek with a shameful "defacto" segregation. Housing and public schools still logically attract the different ethnic groups based on their economics and their culture. This is something that cannot be legislated away. Laws can be passed to enforce changes in behavior. Attitudes will take a little longer.

A glaring gap in prevention is seen in the lack of the mammogram as the key to early breast cancer detection and, therefore, potential cure. Although the female breast is the number-one source of all female cancers, the mortality rate from breast cancer is way down on the list. That is certainly due, in part, to mammogram screening, early diagnosis, and treatment. Of the over 200,000 new cases expected each year, less than a quarter will be fatal.

There are two principle causes for that still unacceptably high number, knowing that the disease is containable. One is that when women get lopped off the Medicaid rolls, lose their job perks, or cannot take on a COBRA plan, the mammogram gets sacrificed for food, the rent, the roof repair, or even the kids' goodies under the Christmas tree.

A Kaiser Foundation report again is telltale. A 2004 telephone survey of almost 3,000 women over eighteen showed that mammograms and prescription drugs were skipped first when hard times hit. Less than half of the eligible women in the country who are uninsured will have their annual PAP smear and mammogram. It has been shown that women (56 percent) are more likely than men (42 percent) to use prescription drugs on a regular basis, and they are tragically more likely to drop those needed meds due to financial crunches.

The second cause is uneven physician distribution. The best definition of conservatism is the simple one—just wanting to keep the status quo. Conservatives like things the way they are. The United States has always prided itself in maintaining that status quo when it comes to free enterprise and boasts of the American model that allows for graduating hospital residents to go wherever they want to start their careers as private practitioners.

That ends up with many regions in the country going without adequate physician services. That over 300:1 ratio that is a national average of people to doctor is grossly distorted because of our erratic distribution. In major urban centers, outside their ghettos, the 180:1 optimal ratio is easily met and then some.

But in the rural South and West or even in the parts of the Eastern corridor with a rigorous topography, doctors are sometimes hard to come by. Patients understandably shy away from the expense and ardor of long travel, especially for those vital check-ups, preventive visits, and needed follow-ups. This is more so for senior citizens, who often are thus not able to take advantage of their Medicare benefits.

The economic upturn of the 1990s did bring about some improvement in healthcare throughout the nation. It was not a dramatic increase and in no way suggested that total coverage was around the corner. It was more of a trickle-down effect, something like Presidents Ronald Reagan and George H. Bush promised us by their tax cuts for the rich and famous, that predicted "supply side" benefit. We are still waiting.

But as we slid back into the doldrums of the economic downturn at the turn of the millennium, the nation became more aware of its old nemesis—racism. And just as wage gaps get wider every year between men and women and whites and blacks, so does their healthcare status. Those black and white gaps can only be called dramatic.

Examples abound. The most glaring is the AIDS epidemic of the 1980s and 1990s. After its etiology was confirmed and the gay population altered its behavior to just about eliminate new cases, the HIV syndrome filtered down almost exclusively to the dirty needle intravenous drug users, disproportionately black and Latino.

Allocations were announced in Washington; only a small fraction ever got down to the trenches.

Perinatal and neonatal mortality, those sometimes-still-observed gold standards that mark the quality of healthcare of a people, especially in the developed nations, still indicate a most shameful disparity between the different ethnic groups. U.S. blacks die at twice the rate of U.S. whites of diabetes, hypertension, and AIDS. Tuberculosis at many times the rate. Sexually transmitted disease also shows at least a six times difference between whites and those of color.

The mystery is why anyone thinks the reasons are mysterious. Without that precious, ubiquitous, and elusive healthcare program that would obey the "separate and equal" rule, the social and medical causes of the disparity are there for all to see. Show me an authority that says the reasons are unknown or "mysterious," and I will show you either a racist or a fool.

Or both.

The Vulnerable Group: Our Children

Let no child be left behind. Sound familiar? That smacks of another White House bit of advice another era ago—Just Say No! Both adages are as shallow as they sound. These Oval Office sound bites talked the talk but never walked the walk.

A fifth arm of the HCFA is the federally financed State Children Health Insurance Program (SCHIP) that is yet another band-aid for those 45 million without any healthcare protection. The harsh reality is that just as Washington is poised to launch an attack on Medicaid and Medicare, the nation's youth will not be spared.

When CHIP was enacted in 1997, there were 10 million children without health insurance. Closing in on a decade later, more than one-third still go without even the excuse we call public health insurance—Medicaid.

A 2005 University of California research project noted that half of the state's poorest children settled for publicly funded healthcare programs (Medicaid) but that as the announced Bush Medicaid cuts go into effect over the next five years, by 2010, over 20 percent of the children will be without any coverage whatsoever. The Bush II entitlement cuts that started out with that $10 billion from Medicaid include a reversion of $2.8 million each year to the U.S. Treasury from previously designated funds that were bound for SCHIP.

The PR out of Washington is careful to clamor that No Child Left Behind is for real and any curtailments planned for healthcare are being wary of the needs of children. It is obvious that as the American public is being sold on tax cuts for the wealthy and supply side economics, slashes in Medicaid maybe can be sneaked past the people, but not our children. The Administration knows that such insensitivity would never get by.

"Honest" Abe told us that you can fool all of the people some of the time or some of the people all of the time. But you can never fool all of the people all of the time.

Class and Race

This boils down to the demographics that cover it all and say it all. Economics.

Just as Washington told the fiscally troubled people of New York City an era or two ago to DROP DEAD in a major daily tabloid headline that probably cost the incumbent the state's electoral votes and the White House, it appears that same message is being handed down from the Oval Office to the poorest of Americans. We didn't need the New Orleans disasters of Hurricanes Katrina and Rita in the fall of 2005 to show us the different ways people of color are handled by our social and governmental structures.

That the Oval Office and Health and Human Services would even toy with that only lifeline for the poor, Medicaid, is showing an insensitivity that goes beyond the pale.

For sure, as expected, healthcare statistics are reflective of the general differences in our widening economic gap. The "gradient effect" applies here. Each socioeconomic group, as measured and defined by social and economic characteristics such as education, literacy, *de facto* living conditions, and income, has better health by all measurements than the one below it. Indeed, education is the most telling correlation. The more schooling, the better the health of any group.

Differences do exist among the races and ethnic groups per se. African-Americans, Latinos, and American Indians suffer from poorer health outcomes compared to white and the general population at any level of income. The poor simply have restricted access to good housing, cleaner air and water, and other environmental states. The impact of psychological factors, such as stress and family stability, and in general, lesser access to whatever healthcare machinery is available but often goes unknown and under utilized by a down-trodden people, adds to their desperation.

Just as that fellow in the ER would not trust that his neighbor's kid could become a cardiologist, many people of a ghetto community have come to mistrust their local clinics run by out-of-neighborhood personnel without strong identification ties. The people never know if they are being shortchanged or perhaps being used as "guinea pigs" for some new drug or experimental treatment procedure. They often are.

Neighborhoods play a huge role. They are important influences on the health of any people having to face higher infant mortality and birth outcomes, stymied child development, less nutritional and sanitation facilities, and decrepit housing, ignoring health-related behaviors, such as mental health. The highest rate of childhood asthma in the country, for example, is in the south Bronx borough in New York City, a socially and economically deprived area with its high incidence of rodent and cockroach infestations. Cause and effect have been clinically and laboratory shown.

Two doctors and an HMO manager had passed on and were lined up together at the Pearly Gates. St. Peter was at the desk to decide on the applicants' merits for entry.

The first physician presented his ID that noted he had been a fine pediatric surgeon. "I mended and saved hundreds of children." St. Peter waved him onward.

The second doctor told of his work as an obstetrician and how he had helped bring so many healthy newborns into the world. The "Pearly Gatekeeper" nodded for him to proceed.

Finally, the HMO manager claimed he had arranged for a countless number of family clients to get cost-effective healthcare. St. Peter mused over the situation and then looked up and said, "You may enter as well, sir, but you can stay only three days. Then you can go to hell." ♦

When I commented earlier that if you think healthcare is expensive, try sickness, it was not tongue-in-cheek. The poor health of the uninsured carries one hell of a price tag.

As the quantity of the uninsured goes up and up in actual numbers as well as a percentage of the population, so do the costs of keeping them around. It has been estimated by more than one actuarial that the price tag for the uncovered is in the more than $100 billion range, give or take a couple of billion either way.

Contrary to myth, this cost is not only to provide healthcare in the public hospitals on the public dole, but from the poor health of the disenfranchised. There are the lost revenues on the factory and the farm and all service industries. Especially service industries where human labor cannot be substituted that easily, if at all, by a robot or mechanized assembly line that has become the cornerstone of the U.S. economy.

There is, of course, that difficult-to-measure intangible loss of productivity from overt absenteeism or when workers anywhere are not at their best. The less-than-optimal working force is more prone to needed rest and, worst of all, accidents on the job.

Like I said. If you think staying healthy is expensive, try sickness.

Journalist Gretchen Cook described over the Internet how her mother met her ill-prepared death and "was ashamed of getting sick."

My mother died of emphysema, Cook wrote. I was there...the image will not go away. She was a heavy smoker and suffered as much from that knowledge as...she did from her painful condition.

I know only too well that shame is a lonely affliction. [She] was not an activist but was able to rail against the tobacco companies that got her addicted...the system that left her so abandoned...Smoking seemed to be her greatest pleasure, one of the few things she was able to control in her life. ♦

Another Vulnerable Group: The Old Folks and the Role of the Doctor-Assisted Suicide (DAS)

The American society average age is increasing rapidly. That is the good news. The bad news is that society will then be suffering with age-related chronic illnesses. More bad news. The number of providers, professional and volunteer, is dwindling. As Medicare gets more convoluted and overwhelmed by subtle changes that affect the daily practice of the clinicians, more and more of them are shying away from accepting any Medicare patients at all.

Isn't it remarkable that a mama or a papa can raise and take care of five or six kids but not one of them can later on take care of one mama or papa? ♦

Euthanasia is a topic that does not seem to go away, like abortion and the death penalty. Many advocate that this is a way of dealing with the problem of the debilitated. As convicted DAS pioneer Dr. Jack Kevorkian sits in his prison cell, there are more and more who are pondering if he did not have the right answer after all.

A 2005 *New York Times* editorial defended "death with dignity," a forefront issue the Supreme Court, with its new justices appointed by a conservative administration led by a born-again Christian right-wing president, will be dealing with these coming next several years. The *Times* noted, seemingly to avoid dogmatism, that we must be sensitive to those who are "likely" to die.

How likely? Very likely? Very, very likely? Just a tad likely? Not so likely tomorrow? Who decides how likely? To disgruntled family members and their contingency-paid attorneys, more likely than yesterday? On what basis? The size of the estate? The wording of the last will and testament? Such editorials always point out that there are those developed nations in the world that have adopted some form of euthanasia, and with apparent success and no regret. So far.

A guy fell from the roof deck of the 104-story Empire State Building in New York City. As he was plummeting past the 55th floor, someone inside yelled out at him, "How are you doing?"

"So far, so good," came the reply. ♦

But what is always avoided is the rest of the story. That those few countries with some form of euthanasia and DAS also have full federal health coverage for their people. With 100 percent doctor coverage, hospital and hospice care, and prescription medications. Without loopholes or co-pays. They have been given every opportunity to live out their lives in dignity, not having been discarded. Nor do they apparently feel discarded, many studies have reported. Therein lies the difference. Until we have given our debilitated citizens the right to live and assure them we have provided the means to do so, regardless of their economic status, we cannot and must not offer them death as an alternative to their infirmities.

This further points out the nature of our healthcare crisis.

The issue of abortion/choice, another topic that continues to haunt the nation's airwaves and courtrooms, is directly entwined with the healthcare debate. For although abortion/choice is certainly and rightfully being contested on legal, moral, social, ethical, and religious grounds, as well as a medical controversy, it is safe to say that much of the steam of the argument would dissipate if the women of America had full healthcare insurance. If the procedure were but an appurtenance of total and secure women's healthcare, it would surely be less in the spotlight and singled out.

Since Roe v Wade is, in essence, a patient and doctor rights and privacy decision, it stands out because so many American women go without healthcare in general. When that landmark 1973 Supreme Court decision accepted the exchange between doctor and patient as such, it became noticed that these women in need are suddenly allowed that access. A good deal of the ensuing debate raged over healthcare's being a form of a privilege, and therefore that privilege could be denied someone when there were those legal, moral, social, ethical, and religious parameters involved.

Every rocket or gun that is fired, every warship launched...signifies a theft from those who are hungry and not fed, cold and not clothed...(ill and not cared for)...This is not a way of life. —President Dwight David Eisenhower, from "The Chance for Peace" address, April 16, 1963. ♦

Clear and Present Danger

As 2006 was looming, the nation was being inundated with the concerns that the Avian flu was perhaps on its way, and, remembering the 1918 epidemic that took over 20 million lives worldwide, maybe 4 million in the USA, we might be in for the long haul again. Might. There is a feeling that the flu scare may just be that, and nowhere near the risk clamored about. That it is instead just another scare to keep our minds off the body bag counts in Iraq, soaring prices at the gas pump, and a stagnant minimum wage. Potential vaccine shortages are predicted. Remember, prevention medications that are far less profitable than therapeutics are not high on the production agenda of the nation's drug houses.

And we only have to shudder at what the country went through, not yet over, with the devastation of Hurricanes Katrina and Rita on the Gulf Coast in the fall of 2005. Without a federally run universal healthcare program, we were in no way prepared for the tide of various maladies and syndromes that were thrown at us by the rushing waters.

Nature is often not kind. Other Katrinas and Ritas are waiting in the wings. Without some form of national health, we will forever be unprepared.

If there's a nuclear terrorist attack or a major pandemic...you're going to see a level of government incompetence that'll take you back to the Declaration of Independence. —Col. Lawrence Wilkerson, Ex-Aide to then-Secretary of State Colin Powell, October 19, 2005. ♦

General Motors is concerned that it will not be able to keep up with other auto maker countries and competition that did not have to allow for as much as $1,500 extra in the production costs of each car to cover employee healthcare. In October 2005, GM managed to get concessions from the United Auto Workers (UAW) Union that had been until then considered unthinkable—an almost quadruple contribution by the workers into their healthcare.

The present 7 percent vigorish paid out by the worker now will shoot up to an unconscionable 27 percent.

That $10 billion slash in Medicaid funding planned by the Bush Administration over the next decade is already bearing fruit, as Washington sees its budgets needing more and more to support the Iraq debacle and whatever other foreign hegemonic adventures it has in store for us.

Starting in the logical state, the president's brother's state of Florida, it has been announced that there will be an immediate and total transformation in its Medicaid program. With children under twenty-one and pregnant women still exempt (read:stay tuned), the state has been given White House approval to limit spending on its 2.2 million beneficiaries, resulting in severe limitations in already abstemious Medicaid services.

Then there is the announcement that a new drug, Herceptin, is being rushed to market because of its amazing and proud success in the management of any and all levels of breast cancer in women. The National Cancer Institute stated that Herceptin was planned to be ready for public use by 2007. But the early clinical trials have been so remarkably positive, it can justify getting the drug out to a suffering population sooner than expected. How about that for some good news?

Now let the other shoe drop. A year's supply of Herceptin will be costing $48,000. I kid you not. That's forty-eight thousand dollars! So much for breast cancer cures. There are other new agents that are also in that price range.

How about this for going in a cuckoo direction? A new breed of privateering is finding a home in the United States. Ergo the birth of the "concierge boutique" doctors. These physicians (please stay calm, Hippocrates) have brought capitation to a new height. For the haves, that is. For an exchange of an annual cash retainer, you have bought yourself a doctor for the year. The bonuses are his/her prime time, unlimited phone calls, 24/7, even a house call if deemed necessary. You get the human physician and all of that office's state-of-the-art electronic surveillance equipment at your disposal and command.

It started sporadically in 1996, as a trial run, and has now taken off. More and more are getting into this practice. Like a "country club for the rich," said Representative Pete Stark (D-CA) in Congress. "The healthcare system will become even more inequitable than it is today." No foolin.'

CHAPTER 11

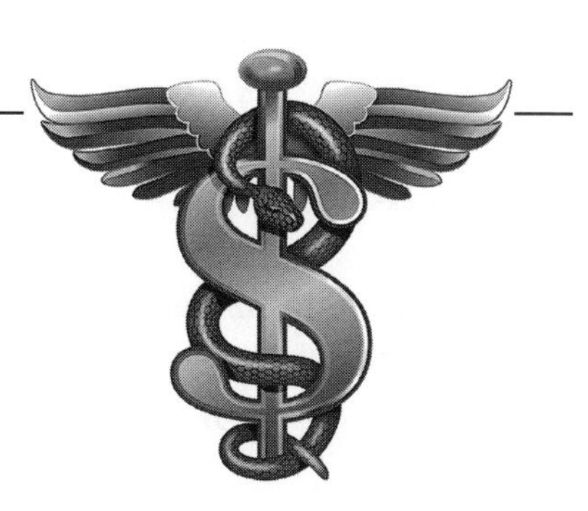

Mending the System: Physician, Heal Thyself

A manufacturer of household items decided what America needed was a new style of mousetrap. The company's marketing team approached the dean of a leading engineering university with its proposal, but with one proviso. The new device had to include a baby grand piano. The professor accepted the challenge, and within the specified time, the creation was unveiled to the public. There were three problems. It was very cumbersome, it was very expensive, and it did not trap any mice. ♦

From all of this rubble, I proffer three solutions to relieve this healthcare morass in the United States of America that demands our attention and action.

One. That the health of a people must be reclassified and defined. Healthcare is not a privilege. It is a right. A right of all living souls in this world. No exceptions. Deny them healthcare and you deny them that right. They are disavowed the very fabric of life. The United States has never adopted a social policy that has included healthcare in that context.

Right (rīt) n: Something that is morally, ethically, and legally proper; that which is just and good; endowed by nature.
–Merriam-Webster's Collegiate Dictionary ♦

We flirted with it in the first of FDR's New Deal administrations and settled. The Great Society of LBJ then and since led to our most memorable breakthrough, with an advancement—Medicare—that has been among the greatest accomplishments in our history. But that is still far from enough. Throughout the whole discussion of the controversy, healthcare has always been looked upon as a privilege, something that the government was going to offer as a gift. A handout. Never as a right that cannot be denied to the people.

"...everyone has the right to...health and well-being of his/her family, including...medical care...and the right to security in the event of...sickness...or disability." —Universal Declaration of Human Rights, Article 25, UN General Assembly, December 10, 1948. ♦

In 1791, the great revolutionary Thomas Paine issued his *The Rights of Man.* This was in the form of a letter to President George Washington in retort to the criticism of both the American and French revolution, then in its throes.

Paine expressed his passion for human rights, as defined to be born free; to be assured of life, liberty, and the pursuit of happiness, to be free of oppression and from unlawful arrest. This was all in affirmation of the Declaration of Independence of 1776, the Revolution, and the French struggle for freedom from the tyranny of the throne and the bourgeoisie.

In a January 1941 address to Congress, President Franklin D. Roosevelt changed the face of the human rights of man (read: woman, too) forever. The term "Four Freedoms" became a part of our lexicon.

There was the freedom (read: rights) of speech and expression.

The second was the right (read: freedom) for all Americans to worship God in their own way.

The fourth was that precious freedom from fear, which FDR interpreted as a reduction in world armaments and that no nation in the world would commit an act of aggression against any other. Do you think anyone in Washington today has ever read FDR's memo?

The third, deliberately mentioned last, described a freedom from want that FDR translated into world terms, to "secure every nation a *healthy* peacetime life." It is safe to assume the president had been reminded of the need for the people's health by his great confidante, Secretary of Labor Frances Perkins, always at the president's side at significant political moments. This was the very first time in American history that health as an entity and term was mentioned from any official podium as a description of the role of government. Even Tom Paine didn't go that far.

The International Covenant of Economic, Social, and Cultural Rights...called upon government to create "conditions which would assure to all medical service." —UN General Assembly, December 16, 1966 ♦

Two. That the United States of America, in order to protect that right forever, use the inherent machinery for such a guarantee. That there be enacted and passed a twenty-eighth amendment to the U.S. Constitution that would define healthcare as a right for all.

The Constitution, with all its brilliance, is a flawed document. It was conceived, constructed, and construed by a ruling group of white men, property and slave owners all, who put together a set of basic laws for the newly formed nation. It originally provided for no protection of the rights of blacks or women.

The instrument dealt with the formation of a new government, free from the rule of the English throne. It provided for executive, judicial, and legislative branches, put there by a form of a popular vote, but only if you were white, male, and owned a hunk of dirt. The first president of the country was elected by 7 percent of the U.S. population at the time.

But there was not a single word or affirmation that bestowed the means of an education or the health of the people.

Indeed, the first ten amendments (the Bill of Rights) and over the next 200 years the subsequent amendments secured the rights to religion of one's choice; freedom of speech and the press (now anyone with $100 million can start up a newspaper); the right to assemble; the right to form a militia; the principle of habeas corpus; a trial by jury of one's peers; the abolition of slavery; the vote for all without restriction from race, color, previous condition of servitude, and, eventually, sex; the collection of income taxes; the prohibition of alcoholic beverages, and then its repeal; the lowering of voting rights to age eighteen.

The good news is that there is a *modus operandi* for more amendments. The Equal Rights Amendment (ERA) for women didn't fail by too much as recently as 1977. But it will take a commitment that declares healthcare as that right instead of a privilege. It all starts there.

A twenty-eighth amendment is the one way to assure us all of that declaration.

That is also the sure way to declare the denial of healthcare to the American people is a national problem requiring a national solution, for only the U.S. Constitution sets a national standard. When the Supreme Court, charged with interpreting the Constitution, hands down a decision, it automatically covers all fifty states. That is the way it was intended.

Why? National problems require national solutions.

Three. That once healthcare is declared a right and a Constitutional amendment is eventually passed that assures that right be protected forever, that the federal government act to live up to that responsibility as an entitlement, never discretionary.

Five Giant Steps Forward

There are five qualities that are necessary for our nation and its governmental apparatus to assume.

1) That healthcare coverage be comprehensive. There can be no stone uncovered, no leaf unturned, and no human pathology ignored. There is no way to qualify a given human ailment as more significant than any other. There are no two human diseases that are the same. Like your fingerprints or DNA. The same ones, clinically identical, can act totally different in the same patient just moments later.

The human body responds and reacts to a given noxious agent, be it a microorganism, a stress of nature, a genetic or inborn imbalance, a response to a toxic behavior or emotion, or a combination of all of the above, in different ways. The physicians' skills are called upon to possibly predict and then go forward in a preventive manner, always prepared to treat and control when those predictions go awry and run amok.

2) That health coverage must be universal every way. No human being residing in the United States of America can be denied, regardless of race, color, creed, previous condition of servitude, sex, or age. With healthcare a right, no one can be dismissed from the system. No one.

3) That such care be transferable to all fifty states or, for that matter,

wherever and whenever Americans travel abroad. Just as we have come to understand that our rights are protected around the globe, and that we have that sense of security that our embassies act as protectorates of our rights wherever we are, so must we have the security of knowing perhaps our most precious right, healthcare, will always be assured.

4) That such coverage must be available and accessible across the board. No registered, accredited, and licensed healthcare professional or institution of any sort, by statute, can opt out of the system. Their legal permit to practice their trade is automatically national in scope and demands they be available to care for all who seek to be their patients.

5) And finally, to provide the people with their newly declared right to healthcare by skilled practitioners and healthcare professionals and institutions, a National Health Service be inaugurated. This NHS is to be a publicly supported, tax-sustained entitlement, single-payer, fully administered agency of the federal government with cabinet rank, prestige, and empowerment.

Healthcare is just too important to be left in the hands of profit driven and motivated private business interests. It is just that simple, stupid.

This is not pie-in-the-sky thinking. Grass roots protests and activism have turned the government around before. There was the Boston Tea Party, the Martin Luther King, Jr., Washington Mall march, the uproar over Vietnam, and the clamor that brought down the World Trade Organization (WTO) in Seattle.

What then follows is the grass roots activism that would be the machinery for change. Anthropologist Margaret Mead put it this way. "Never doubt," she said, "that a small group of thoughtful committed citizens can change the world. Indeed, it is the only thing that ever has."

Groups throughout the nation, such as *Art Without Walls, Acts of Art, Healthcare-NOW!*, and *Physicians for a National Health Program* (www.pnhp.org), among others, are springing up as we speak. Local offices are opening in just about every major urban center. Check your phonebook or the Internet.

MISSION STATEMENT

WHEREAS, over 45 million U.S. Americans are without any form of healthcare coverage and many tens of millions more are with inadequate care;

WHEREAS, our only existing government/public programs, Medicaid and Medicare, are continually subjected to Administration slashes in funding, services, and personnel;

WHEREAS, the U.S. pharmaceutical industry cost structure leaves numerous, even vital, prescription medicines unaffordable to the many;

WHEREAS, a privatized managed-care system of Health Maintenance Organizations (HMOs) with its excessive profits and bureaucracy has been the government's answer to the country's healthcare needs;

WHEREAS, we remain the world's only developed nation without a total healthcare program for its people;

WE, under the aegis of Healthcare-NOW! or our allied activist organizations, establishing healthcare as a right instead of a privilege, are committed to the following agenda:

THAT a plan be put into effect that is comprehensive, covering all healthcare needs;

THAT it be universal to include everyone living in the United States of America, without exception;

THAT it be accessible throughout the nation with all healthcare professionals bound by law to serve everyone;

THAT it be transferable anywhere in the USA and whenever citizens travel abroad;

THAT it consist of a federally sponsored and administered single-payer program that includes all facilities, personnel, services, and medications;

TO this we pledge all our efforts and resources.

Physicist Max Born's axiom about space travel applies here. Intellect tells us the difference between the possible and the impossible; reason the difference between the sensible and the senseless. HMO managed care is a triumph of intellect but a tragic failure of reason. ♦

One more sobering thought

Our dearth of healthcare is not the enigma many have made it out to be. It is not an isolated link in an otherwise social-justice-sensitive government's thinking. It is part of the chain of foreign and domestic policies that have prompted the rest of the world to perceive us as the world's imperialist villain.

HMO/managed care, as our healthcare delivery system, has been brought to you by the same people who have given us such dubious adventures as Vietnam, Desert Storm, the illegal Cuban blockade, the Nicaraguan campaign, land deal give-a-ways to Big Oil, stem cell research resistance, the Enron collapse and its fallout, presidential wars that found no weapons of mass destruction; abuses at Abu Ghraib and Guantanamo, threats to Roe v Wade, higher and higher military budgets, tax breaks for the wealthy, wire taps without warrants, Deibold manipulations of national elections, stagnation of the minimum wage. And these are just for openers.

Being unhealthy is just too scary a concept to contemplate. It is not acceptable. For without health, there can be no music, science, art, highways, business, ballet, sports, algebra, literature, fun, computers, farming, airplanes, movies, animal rights, cars, books, spaghetti, babies, space exploration, beach umbrellas, rollercoasters, picnics, sex. In a word, life as we know it would not exist.

HMO managed care is that mousetrap with the baby grand piano. It is cumbersome, expensive, and will not take care of those in need.

It is my hope that *Practicing Medicine Without a License* will become the manifesto for the coming revolution in U.S. healthcare. The American people deserve and must settle for nothing else.

Of all the forms of inequality, injustice in healthcare is the most shocking and inhumane. –Reverend Martin Luther King, Jr. ♦

Q&A

Frequently Asked Questions About a National Health Service

Q: Can we as a nation afford a federal NHS? Where will the money come from? Will my taxes go up if there is a national health plan for everyone?
A: We cannot afford not to have a national healthcare plan. The USA is the most affluent of developed nations. Where will the money come from for healthcare? That's easy—from where it is going. New taxes will not be needed.

We will be covered by the funds now expended on Medicaid and Medicare, our two existing federal programs. To this we add what is now being spent on private care, savings from the reduction in administrative overhead, from the present 15 to 20 percent to the expected 3 to 4 percent. It all starts with a single-payer program.

Ben Franklin's adage that an ounce of prevention is worth a pound of cure, holds here.

Q: Is Conyers' HR 676 the answer?
A: Perfect it is not. But then, is anything? HR 676 is our golden parachute. National health demands a national solution. And HR 676 is federal, single-payer, universal, and comprehensive. Just as Medicaid and Medicare showed, national health is possible to pull off. The gaps that give some of the privateers and hospitals a little too much leeway must be slowly eliminated, once we see the plan is viable, workable, affordable, and Congressionally available. It is a great place to start.

Q: How do we get involved in this struggle?
A: Grass roots organizations are springing up all over the place. Citizen and Congressional rallies and hearings are planned. Unions, civic

groups, and medical organizations with nurses and doctors at the helm are there for the joining and contributing. Celebrities are joining the struggle; HR 676 is gaining momentum up on the Hill.

Health Care-NOW! is at the forefront, with offices in New York and throughout the nation: 339 Lafayette St.. New York, NY. 212-475-8350 www.healthcare-now.org.

The artist community is also involved. Contact: Acts of Art at actsart@gmail.com, and Art Without Walls, 165 Clinton Ave. Brooklyn, NY 11205. 718-852-8798.

Q: Since a full healthcare program is so obviously needed and there is no social downside, why has it been so difficult to get it? Why any opposition?

A: Dr. Larry Brown of the Mailman School of Public Health at Columbia University and other healthcare activists have noted that the opposing political forces are just too mired in their traditions. First, as true conservatives, they are the preservers of the status quo and those corporate private insurance carriers and banking moguls want to keep healthcare as a profit-making business. They are very driven, well organized, and amply financed. Their entrenchment in our social order gives them the edge as the incumbent.

As Maggie Mahar says in *Money-Driven Medicine: The Real Reason Healthcare Costs So Much,* "A professional, the physician pledged to put his patients' interests ahead of his own. The corporation, by contrast, is legally bound to put its shareholders' interests first."

Secondly, the pro-healthcare program movement is fragmented and needs to unify its message and mission. Various states and their politically ambitious governors are presenting their own individual agendas, as though any state could even begin to accomplish such a humongous thing as providing healthcare for their people. Many unions and other community and special interest groups have some semblance of healthcare for their rank and file and use that as a selling point to entice workers and prospective members. Some political figures and elected officials feel their individual programs are the best and end up competing with each other.

There are also those existing proud American "safety nets" that have been sold to the public as a sufficient way of providing healthcare for all in times of need. People in the healthcare trade are generally sensitive to their patients' urgencies and don't like turning anyone away. The nation's public health hospitals, veterans' hospitals, and other such facilities run by local governments are physically available and nonprofit and give the impression that their stop-gap resources are enough. But they fall short of adequately serving the public need. Healthcare is more than putting that proverbial Band-Aid on a hemorrhage. It needs what only a true national program can provide.

Q: What will become of the insurance carriers?
A: As the melody goes, somethin's gotta give. There is no place for private industry and profit-aiming corporations in our healthcare system. Health, along with education, is just too important to be left up to the privateers whose financial gains usually take priority over the success of their products. Healthcare is too vital and humongous to continue to throw away that extra 15 percent on profits and wasteful bureaucracy.

There is precedent. The public utilities, although not entirely public, were created because it was deemed that certain services, like power and communication, were too vital not to have some form of strict governmental control. When the privately held utility companies refused to provide the Southeast U.S. with electric power in the throes of the Great Depression, the feds stepped in, created the Tennessee Valley Authority (TVA), and proved again that federal programs can be successful.

Yes, we can all expect to be barraged with promo ads by the private carriers that it is downright un-American to take away from our private entrepreneurs. But the U.S. Constitution is clear, if not specific. The public good comes first. We allow for and confiscate land and property when highways and public security services are needed. The TVA is the visible program. Others abound.

Q: How does a Constitutional amendment get passed?
A: Article V of the U.S. Constitution explains this process. In Congress, whenever two-thirds of both Houses vote in favor of a member's proposed amendment, it goes to both floors for debate and also on to every state legislature for open discussion. It then comes to a final balloting and is deemed valid and added to the amendment section

of the Constitution after three-quarters of the state legislatures or a drawn Constitutional convention votes in its favor. It then becomes the law of the land.

There is sufficient precedent for such an action. The original ten amendments passed in 1787 are called, as we know, the Bill of Rights. Others have been proposed, for such things as voting rights, executive succession, slavery abolition, etc. The last amendment, Number 27, was a Congressional pay regulation passed in 1992. The Equal Rights Amendment (ERA) got its thirty-seventh state legislature vote in 1992, but never got the required thirty-eighth, and it failed.

Q: What will be the role of the states?
A: Depends on where you start. Medicaid now has state regulatory offices, with all financing, of course, coming from Washington. Just about all states have varied administrative rules and regulations, approved by the national office. The same goes for their budgets and how the individual state spends its federal allocation. State Medicaid is also moving the way the nation did back in 1993—toward privately run HMO machinery.

Medicare, on the other hand, is strictly federal, and for that reason, Medicare-for-all has been considered by many a logical way to begin the NHS process. That would only be acceptable if the kinks in the Medicare program were ironed out. Like assuring that all healthcare facilities and personnel were part of the process, and all enrollees were eligible for total care. That is not so now, in that many physicians have opted out of the system and simply chosen not to participate.

Conyers' HR 676 does establish regional state units, replacing Medicare offices and personnel in most cases. But it also details that each state office and administrator is to report to a national center for federal administration and quality control.

Q: Will all hospitals take anyone in need?
A: They'd better. That would be the law. A national health service is just that—national. No healthcare facility would be licensed to operate unless it agrees to get with the program.

Q: Will there be payment if the services provided are inadequate? How about abuse of the system?
A: What would a system be without abusers? Nonexistent or a lie. Of

course any system can expect in-house abusers. But like every other national system in the entire developed world, and the federal systems now in operation, watchdog groups would have to do their jobs to keep abuse at a minimum. That goes for both providers and enrollees.

That is surely a good reason for having a federal system for our healthcare. Only the feds have been shown to adequately police themselves.

Q: How about paperwork? Who files claims?
A: The federal machinery would easily solve this problem, just as is done now in Medicaid and Medicare and the HR 676 proposal. Standardized, office-generated claims go to a single payment center. All medical service centers would have the same rules and regulations. That is why overhead with single-payer is minimal, throughout the world and with U.S. Medicare. KISS keep it simple, stupid.

As the claims become standard and, of course, electronically generated, the system will be easier to follow and will run smoothly. As it stands now, private carriers have gatekeepers, watchdogs, overseers, and monitors galore, all adding to the costs of the services and the time it takes to wend your way through. But with an NHS, there will be no more doctors jockeying with the HMO offices or negotiations for a better return. And the terms and conditions of treatment, coverage, and payment will not change as they do now.

Patients would not file claims. Offices with trained personnel would. KISS.

Q: What will happen to Medicaid and Medicare if a true NHS comes into effect?
A: They would be easily absorbed into the system. Their administrations and experiences would be borrowed to avoid the pitfalls and capture the successes. Why not? There would be a national, combined Medicaid and Medicare that would include those tens of millions of Americans who go without coverage. We would just give it a new name.

Q: What will happen if there is an epidemic that rocks the nation?
A: A national health service, just as Medicaid has allegedly done for the poor and Medicare for the elderly, would eventually take hold and become a secure avenue for care, just as it is in England, Canada, and the other countries in the industrialized world.

Epidemics and shocks to our people that demand healthcare, like diseases and natural disasters of all sorts, now cause a panic because the people do not trust our healthcare delivery system. And for good reason. There is none to depend on. The events of recent years, from waves of worldwide diseases from abroad to Katrinas and Ritas to 9/11 have taught us, or should have, that only an NHS would give people the needed feeling of safety.

Q: Suppose I move from one state to another. Or get sick or injured when I travel abroad. Covered?
A: A dictum of national health includes portability and accessibility. Every covered U.S. citizen is just that—covered no matter where travels take him or her. That is a main advantage of national health—it is national. International, when called for.

That would go as well for your employment or family status. An NHS would never be dependent on your family size, your age, or your employment. You are not covered because of your personnel office. You are covered because you are an American.

Q: Are specialists, all services, and tests included and covered? Do I have a choice of doctor and facility?
A: Universality is a mainstay of a proposed NHS. All licensed doctors, healthcare professionals, and facilities are automatically a part of the program. No one can opt out. No patient can be denied. No legitimate medical service can be eliminated.

Q: Are there any hidden costs out-of-pocket?
A: Absolutely not. That is one way to reduce bureaucracy. All services are covered; all services are paid for. KISS.

Q: Are aliens covered?
A: Yes. All U.S. citizens are entitled by accident of birth to be covered. But for emergent/urgent care, aliens who essentially are our guests until given either citizen status or whatever their choice, are included in the coverage. Remember, sickness drains all of us. It makes no fiscal or social sense to ignore the needy.

Q: Who has access to medical records in an NHS?

A: Those who need to access them in order to provide optimal care. Profit-minded carriers are competing for patients while seeking to avoid covering individuals with pre-existing conditions that they claim drain their facilities and funds. Under a single-payer, federal program, healthcare would be under one, giant umbrella, "Pre-existing conditions" would never become an issue.

Q: Are there any death benefits under such a plan?
A: Just as Medicare covers death benefits minimally, an NHS would, as well.

Q: Suppose a doctor or service commits a negligence. What will be my redress?
A: Medical malpractice is currently a growth industry. But the defense costs add enormously to the price of healthcare.

Part of this is definitely because of the medical industry, via HMOs. Their private doctors/providers are looked upon as profit-seeking service deliverers. Starting frivolous legal actions becomes part of the game.

Under a system where the people understand their doctors are nicely rewarded tradespeople whose motive is patient care and not profit, the whole psyche of med-mal changes, as it has everywhere else.

While your options for redress are still available, the major changes in the entire profile of not-for-profit healthcare will likely diminish the litigious state of affairs medicine has become today, to be almost non-existent—as it is in every other country with an NHS. So, med-mal attorneys, along with private healthcare insurance carrier agents, would have to look for another day job.

Q: Do we have enough doctors and other personnel if everyone is covered in full?
A: Yes, and maybe, no. With our private practice system, and this being who and what we are, doctors and anyone else can come and go as they please. So as expected, medical meccas and centers and empires have more than enough personnel, leaving America's hinterlands in need. Distribution is the key. That 180:1 optimal ratio of people to doctor is a long way off yet. We stand at about 320:1 overall.

It is logical to assume that with a national health service, the *modus operandi* could and would be able to assign doctors throughout the country, so as to equalize that ratio a little better until we can create and operate more medical schools. But certainly, without question, our present practicing clinicians would be able to handle the patient catchment load until they get relief.

Yes, we would need to train more healthcare personnel. That would fall into place as a national program took hold.

REFERENCES

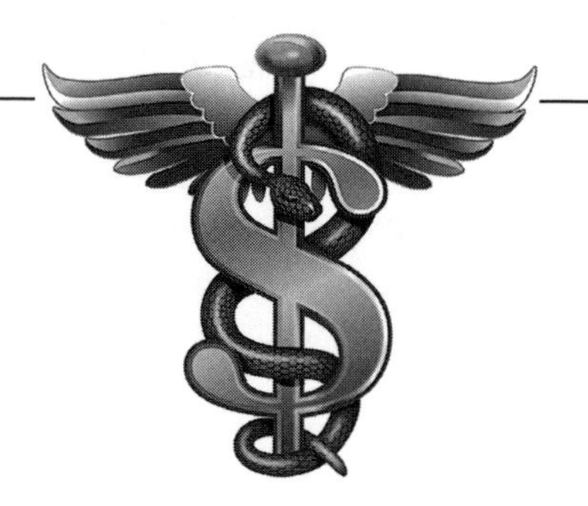

Chapter 1

Case file, patient BL (pseudonym JR) Don Sloan, MD, 1993–6.

Chapter 2

Benjamin, Phil. "National Health and Safety," *People's Weekly World*, 1 May 2004, 10.

Centers for Disease Control, Report 2004. *Data Watch.*

Doyle, Robert. "Health Care Costs. By the Numbers," *Scientific American* 1999: 36.

Garson, Tom. "Death of a Salesman," *The Village Voice*, 26 June 2004. www.villagevoice.com.

Glasser MD, Ronald. "We Are Not Immune," *Harper's Magazine*, March 2006, 35–42.

Halstead, Ted. "The American Paradox," *The Atlantic Monthly* 38(2003): 123–25.

"Health Care in Crisis, A Report," www.dnc002J500smailer.democrat.org. (Accessed 13 March 2003).

Hitti, Miranda. "U.S. Life Expectancy Best Ever," *The CDC Report*, www.wenbm.com/content/Article/101. (Accessed 28 February 2005).

Lopez, Alfedo. "The Iraq Constitution Guarantees Health Insurance," alfredo@people-link.net. (Accessed 4 September 2005).

Marriner, Joanne. "Profit Margins and Mortality," www.Reatesa.AlterNet.org/storyID_17281. (Accessed 1 December 2003).

Mercola MD, Joseph. "Doctors Are the Third Leading Cause of U.S. Patient Deaths," www.mercola.com/2000/jul/30/2000.

Mullan, Fitzhugh . "Physician Brain Drain," *The Atlantic Monthly* 62 (2006): 52.

"The Nation in Numbers. Moral Justice," *The Atlantic Monthly* 39 (2003).

NYC Vital Signs. The State of New York City Health. Vol.2, no. 8:1–11.

Sanders, Representative Bernie. "Time to Consent," *In These Times*, October 2004, 14.

Pear, Robert . "States Forfeit Health Care for Poor Children," *New York Times*, 25 September 2001, national edition.

UNICEF Report, *The Plight of the World's Children, The State of the World's Children* (New York: Oxford University Press), 2001–5.

UNICEF, "State of the World's Children," *NY Transfer News Service* (2005).

UN Report, "Vital Signs," *The Nation*, 11 September 1995, 234.

"Vital Signs," *OB/GYN News* 4 (2004): 6, under Elsevier Publishing, Kaiser Family Foundation. webmaster@kff.org.

Chapter 3

Charman, Karen. "Seeds of Destruction", www.alternet.org/story.html.

Lipoff, Jules. "Med School Confidentia," The *Village Voice*, August 2004, 4–10.

Miller MD, Charles. "The Electronic Medical Record: Is It For You?" *Contemporary OB/GYN* April (2004): 47–53.

Office of Inspector General for Public Affairs, "Compliance Program for Physician Practices," news release, 7 June 2000, 1–2.

Pear, Robert. "Inept Physicians Are Rarely Listed," *New York Times*, 5 August 2001, national edition.

Staff, "Data Watch: Physicians Making Policy," *American Medical Association*. Reprint, *OBGYN News* (2005): 16.

William Whitney Jr. MD, William. "In Health Care, Class Counts. The Nation's Health and Safety," *People's Weekly World*, 28 August 2004, 1–11.

"Who We Are," *Committee of Interns and Residents Bulletin* (February 2005). www.cirseiu.org/ourlocal/cfm.

"Vital Signs," *ObGyn Residents and Training Programs, OBGYN News*, Elsevier International News Group, 10 August 2004.

Chapter 4

Altmeyer, Arthur J. *The Formative Years of Social Security* (University of Madison: Wisconsin Press, 1966).

Brenner, MD, Jos. "The FTAA–Health Hazard for the Americas? Hearing on Public Health Accountability," Center for Policy Analysis, Miami, FL. www.cpath@cpath.org. (Accessed 19 November 2003).

Coming, Peter. 1966. Oral History Interview with Arthur J. Altmeyer. March 23. Washington, DC. www.ssa.guv/history/ajaoral2.html.

"Constructing a Post War World," The GI Roundtable Series in Context. www.historians.org/projects/GIRoundtable.

Doak, Richard. "Drop Loaded 'socialized medicine' Label from the Debate," *Des Moines Register,* 18–19 December 2005. www.desmoinesregister.com.

Skoopol, Theda and Edwin Aments. "Did Capitalists Shape Social Security?" *American Sociological Review* 50:4 (August 1985): 572–75.

Zinn, Howard. *A People's History of the United States* (Harper Perennial, 2000).

CHAPTER 5

Barr, Stephanie. "Hundreds Have Been Hired to Provide New Medicare Drug Benefit," *Washington Post,* 6 April 2005.

Bazie, Michelle. "New Study Finds Rapidly Rising Out-of-Pocket Health Care Cost," *Daybook,* 26 May 2005.

Benjamin, Phil. "Seniors With Medicare Get Short Changed," *People's Weekly World,* 14 January 2001, 15.

Brogan, Pamela. "Medicaid Cuts Only Shift Costs," Gannet News Service, 6 April 2005.

"CDC Data Show That Millions Forgo Needed Treatment," Robert Johnson Foundation Survey, 2 May 2005. www.yubanet.com.

Connolly, Ceci. "Medicare Payments to Doctors Up 15%," *Washington Post,* 1 April 2005. www.washingtonpost.com.

Centers for Medicaid and Medicare Services, *History of Medicaid and Medicare,* 29 January 2005.

Dembner, Alice. "Troubles Foreseen in Medicare's New Rules," *Boston Globe,* 25 April 2005.

"The Drug-Bill Horror Show," *Labor Party Press* 9:1(2004).

"Facts, Myths on Medicaid," *Albany (NY), Times Union,* 10 April 2005.

First United American Life Insurance Company, "Medicare Part D," 12 October 2005.

Gerber, Alex. "Junk Medicaid," *Washington Times,* 29 January 2006, city edition.

Health Care Financing Administration Bulletin, *Medicare and You. Your Medicare Benefits*, 2000–ff.

Hidden Fees of HSAs. PRWEB Bulletin, 25 May 2005.

Hinden, Stan. "Medicare's Part D as Plan B," *Washington Post*, 13 November 2005, regular edition.

Holland, Gina. "High Court Won't Hear Cheaper Drug Cases," Associated Press, 11 October 2005.

Hollis, Mark. "House Approves Medicaid Changes That Would Hit the Poor," *Sun-Sentinel Tallahassee Bureau*, 2 May 2005.

Iglehart, John K. "The American Health Care System-Medicaid," *New England Journal of Medicine* 340:5 (1999): 1–7.

Insurance Carrier Audits and Record Demands. HEP Law. Health Law Education for Professionals. Vol 2, Issue 1 (2005).

Lieberman,Trudy. "Part D From Outer Space," *The Nation*, 30 January 2006, 17–19.

Lubell, Jennifer. "Medicare Fee Cut in Effect Until Congress Returns," *OB-GYN News*, January (2006).

Mazza, Jerry. "New Medicare Law to Clawback Billions for the State," *The Online Journal*, 6 April 2005.

Mallon, Will. "What is Medicare?" *George Mason University Journal*, 29 January 2005.

McCormick, Erin. "Defrauding Medicare," *San Francisco Chronicle*, 18 May 2005.

"Medicaid Could Cost You," CBS News File, 30 March 2005. www.cbsnews.com.

"Medicaid in the Cross Hairs," *New York Times*, 15 March 2005, national edition.

"The Medicare Drug Mess," *New York Times*, 22 January 2006, national edition.

"Medicaid Helping Schools Trim Funding Shortages," *Milwaukee Journal Sentinel*, 5 May 2005, 16.

Moberg, David. "Got Drugs?" *In These Times*, 22 January 2004, 22–24.

Pear, David. "House Approves a Medicare Prescription Benefit," *New York Times*, 28 June 2005, national edition.

Pear, Robert. "Million Parents Lost Medicaid," *New York Times*, 19 June 2005, national edition.

Pear, Robert. "Premium for Medicare Increasing 13%," *New York Times*, 17 September 2005, national report.

Petery, Louis. "Privatizing Medicaid May Out Profits Before People," *My View*. Florida Pediatric Society, 2005.

Pérez-Peña, Richard. "22 States Limiting Doctors' Latitude in Medicaid Drugs," *New York Times*, 16 June 2003, national edition.

Press Associates, Union News Service, "The Prescription Drug Law Rip-off," *People's Weekly World*, 5 November 2005.

Richman, Louis. "Medicaid's Code Red," *New York Times*, 2 October 2005.

Rosen, BS. "Medicare For All!" *People's Weekly World* (Chicago), June 2005, 16.

Roth, Bennett. "Texas Closely Watching Medicaid Budget Battle," *Houston Chronicle*, 10 April 2005.

Salganik, William. "Impact of Drug Benefits Unclear," *The Baltimore Sun*, 1 January 2006. bill.salganik@baltsun.com.

Samuelson, Robert J. "AARP's America Is a Mirage Via AARP Exec Director William Novelli," *AARP Journal*, 16 November 2005.

Saul, Stephanie. "Another Choice for the Elderly: Charity or Medicare?" *New York Times*, 7 November 2005, national edition.

Sullivan, Kip. "Health Scare," *In These Times*, 8 December 2003, 4.

Sullivan, Kip. "Privatizing Medicare," *Z Magazine*, September 2003, 14–16.

Thistle, Scott. "Panel Seeks Curbs on Health Care Costs," *St. Paul News Tribune*, 19 April 2005.

Thomasson, Dan. "Medicaid, Medicare Costs Out of Control," Scripps Howard News Service, 24 July 2005.

Von Hoffman, Nicholas. "Another Case of Torture: The Bush Drug Program," *NY Observer*, 15 November 2005, 4.

Weisman, Joseph. "Report Emphasizes Shortfall in Medicare," *Washington Post*, 24 March 2005. www.washingtonpost.com.

What is EPIC? www.health.state.ny.us/health_care.htm.

Wolf, Richard. "Medicare Prescription Drug Plan Stumps Seniors," *USA Today*, 4 October 2005, national editon.

Wright, Karl. "Next on the Chopping Block: Medicaid," *The Progressive*, 28 January 2004, 28–32.

Chapter 6

Centers for Medicare and Medicaid Services, *HIPAA, The Heath Insurance Portability and Accountability Act of 1996*. www.ems.hhs.gov/hipaa. (Accessed 15 May 2005).

City of New York, Department of Health and Mental Hygiene, *Bulletin,* 27 May 2003.

Elements of the American Health Security Act, Atlanta Journal-Constitution. www.ajc.com/today/content/epapereditions/today/news34c09175043fd0d0.html.

Elswick, Jill. "U.S. Employers Embrace European Rx Model," *Employee News Benefit,* May 2005. www.benefitnews.com.

Fishman, Steve. "Will Operate For Food," *NYMetro,* 6 August 2001. www.nymetro.com.

"Health Insurance for Kids," *San Francisco Chronicle,* 2 May 2005.

"HIPAA Privacy Notice." *St. Barnabas Hospital (2005)*: s1–4.

Jansen, Bart. "Federal Official Gives Maine Rx a Boost," *Portland (Maine) Press Herald,* 1 June 2002.

Snow-Landa, Amy. "Jackson Hole Group Hopes to Spark A Reform Revival," 10 June 2002. www.amednews.com.

Levy, Marc. "Health Care Industry Reported Most in Lobbyist Spending," AP Wire Service, 11 April 2005.

Lionkous, Jeff. "NJ Eyes Savings by Having Health-Conscious Work Force," AP Wire Service, 24 April 2005.

"Paying For Health Care," *Bangor Daily News,* 17 May 2005.

Pear, Robert. "Court Expands the Rights of Patients to Sue HMOs," *New York Times,* 18 February 2003, national edition.

Ropes and Gray, *"Privacy Under HIPAA. What You Need To Know,"* PR Web, March 2003. www.complianced@lenoxhill.net.

Sanders, Representative Bernie. "Time to Consent," *In These Times,* October 2004, 14.

Solomon, Norman. "Why Pretend that Hillary Clinton is Progressive?" *The Huffington Post,* 12 June 2005. www.huffingtonpost.com/norman/solomon/why-pretend-that-hillary- b 22841.html.

Sherman Antitrust Act. www.en.wikipedia.org/wiki/Sherman_Antitrust_act. (Accessed 9 July 2006).

U.S. Department of Labor, Employee Benefits Bulletin, *Questions about COBRA,* April 2005. www.dod.gov/ebsa/faqs/faq.

U.S. Department of Labor Bulletin, *Health Plans and Benefits, COBRA,* 26 April 2005. www.do.1.gov/dol/topic/health.

WHO statement, *World Health on Canada's Proposed Legislative Changes,* issued November 7, 2003. www.padeyg@who.int.

Winokur, Julie. "Live Sicker, Die Younger," *Bulletin*, 15 May 2003. www.aternet.org/story.html.

Woolhandler, MD, Stephanie and David Himmelstein, MD. "Cure a Sick Healthcare System," *In These Times*, 6 August 2004, 32–ff.

World Business Report. www.news.bbc.co.uk/2/hi.

CHAPTER 7

Angell, MD, Marcia. *The Truth About Drug Companies-How They Deceive Us and What to Do About It* (New York: Random House, 2004).

Baker, Dean. "The Real Drug Crisis," *In These Times*, 22 August 1999, 19–21.

Barnett, Antony. "Guardian Public Affairs," 7 December 2003. www.od1tm1.od.nih.gov.

Direct-to-Consumers Advertising and Marketing. www.sireninteractive.com/pdf/pmnews3 10xiov.pdf.

Connolly, Cecil. "Drug Benefit Disparities Accessed," *Washington Post*, 19 April 2005.

Dunn, Jeff. "Breast Cancer Drug Hailed," Associated Press Release, 30 October 2005.

Ezzell, Carol. "The Price of Pills," *Scientific American*, July 2003, 25–35. www.sciam.com.

"FDA Chronology," *Contemporary Ob/Gyn* July (1987): 97–99.

Freudenheim, Milt. "To Promote a New Drug Benefit, Marketers Use Old Scripts," *New York Times*, 3 October 2005, national edition.

Frosch, Dan. "Drug Store Cowboys," 16 November 2004. www.alternet.org.

Gadboury, Fred. "Pharmaceutical Industry, Rx for Profit," *People's Weekly World*, 22 December 2001, 8–12.

Harris, Gardiner. "As Doctor Writes Prescription, Drug Company Writes a Check," *New York Times*, 27 June 2004.

Harris, Gardner. "Drug Firms, Stymied in the Lab, Become Marketing Machines," *Wall Street Journal*, 6 July 2000.

"Generic Drugs Could Save Americans Billions," *Health Day News*, 26 October 2005.

Hilts, Philip J. *Protecting America's Health: The FDA, Business, and One Hundred Years of Regulation* (New York: Alfred Knopf, 1992).

Huffington, Ariana. "Has the Patent Expired on the Pharmaceutical Industry's Invincibility?" 21 May 2002. www.alternet.org/story.html.

Milliman in the Media. www.milliman.com/about_milliman/in-the-news.php.

Millman, Inc. Seattle, Washington, *Millman Report on Health Care Costs*, www.Millman.com. (Accessed 26 May 2005).

Monkerud, Don. "Dealing in Death: Bush's FDA," *Z Magazine*, January 2005, 10.

Moreno-Gonzalez, John. "A Remedy for Drug Price Disparities?" *Newsday*, 19 April 2005, Albany Bureau, 1–2.

Moynihan, Ray and Alan Cassels. "A Disease for Every Pill," *The Nation*, 17 October 2005, 22–25.

Mundy, Alicia. "Hot Flashes Cured by Cold Cash," *Washington Monthly*, 23 January 2003. www.alternet.org.

Murray, Shailagh. "Drug Companies Are Spending Record Amounts on Lobbying," *Wall Street Journal*, 7 July 2000.

National Institutes of Health, *R&D Reports*. www.nih.gov/about/researchresultsforthepublic/index.html. (Accessed 1 July 2006).

Pollitt, Kathryn. "The Moral Property of Women," *The Nation*, 10 July 2000, 9.

Sanders, Representative Bernie. "Can Congress Kick Its Habit? Capital Ideas," *In These Times*, 16 October 2000, 11–12.

Scherer, Michael. "The Side Effects of the Truth," *Mother Jones*, May/June 2003, 71–75.

Shah, Sonia. "Global Clinical Research," *The Nation*, 1 July 2002, 23–25.

Smith, Jeffrey. "Genetically Modified Foods are Inherently Unsafe." www.seedsofdecption.com.

Sullivan, Kip. "Drugs for Vouchers," *Z Magazine*, September 2001, 33–35.

Washburn, Jennifer. "Tainted to the Core," *In These Times*, 20 June 2005, 28–30.

Weisbrot, Mark. "The Cost of Protectionism in Pharmaceuticals," 31 October 2002. www.alternet.com.

Chapter 8

Abelson, Reed. "Whistle-Blower Suit Says Device Maker Generously Awards Doctors," *New York Times*, 24 January 2006, national edition.

Blumenthal, MD, David. "Unhealthy Hospitals," *Harvard Magazine* March/April (2001): 291.

CAPC Manual, *Financing Community Hospitals*, 30 May 2005.

Cropper, Carol Marie. "Consumer Action. Missives from the HMO Battlefield." 20 September 2000. www.smartmoney.com.

Dalrymple, Mary. "Congress Examines Nonprofit Hospitals," Associated Press, 26 May 2005.

Editorial staff. "Amerigroup, One of Country's Best Managed Companies," *Forbes*, 6 June 2005. www.amerigroup.corp.com.

Ehrenreich, Barbara. "The Flip Side. Gouging the Poor," *The Progressive*, 12 February 2004, 12–14.

Facts About the Joint Commission, 6 June 2005. www.jcaho.org/about+us/jcaho.

Gingrich, Newt. "Don't Let Doctors Rig the Market for Specialty Hospitals," *The Internet Journal*, November (2005): A25.

Godon, Suzanne and Timothy McCall, MD. "Healing in a Hurry: Hospitals in the Managed-Care Age," *The Nation*, 1 March 1999, 11–15.

Goldstein, Amy. "Bush to Propose Wider Deductions," *Washington Post*, 25 January 2006.

Graham, Judith. "Needy Patients Find Door Shut When Searching for Specialists," *Chicago Tribune*, 16 May 2005.

Guadagnino PhD, Christopher. "Community Hospital Strategy. Join a Tertiary Hospital Network," *Physician's News Digest*, September (1997): 20.

Kowalczyk, Liz. "Hospitals Study When to Apologize to Patients," *Boston Globe*, 24 July 2005.

"Managed Care, New York's Largest PPOs," *Crains*, 31 August 1998, 4.

Meier, Barry. "Hospital Products Get Seal of Approval," *New York Times*, 23 April 2002, Health Section, national edition.

"Message to the Congress on Proposed Health Care Incentives," *Center for Medicaid and Medicare Services Bulletin*, 28 February 1983.

Shear, Jeff. "Drug Deals. Especially Interested," *Mother Jones*, 3 June 2005, 1–6.

Sullivan, Kip. "Patients Losing Patience," *In These Times*, 20 August 2001, 10.

"Uninsured Get More Discount," *The Milwaukee Journal*, 5 May 2005.

Weiss, Lawrence. *Private Medicine and Public Health* (Westview Press, 1997). Company Profiles on Hospital and Medical Service Plans, Goliath Profiles. www.goliath.ecnext.com/coms2/browse. (Accessed 6 June 2005).

Weissman PhD, Joel. "The Trouble With Uncompensated Hospital Care Perspective," *New England Journal of Medicine*, March (2005): 171–173.

Yen, Hope. "Audit Finds Accounting Flaws at VA. GAO Report on VA Budget," Associated Press, 6 February 2006. www.chroun.com/disp/stm.MP.

CHAPTER 9

Abelson, Reed. "Study Ties Bankruptcy to Medical Bills," *New York Times*, 2 February 2005, national edition.

Angell, Marcia, MD. "Patients' Rights and Other 'Futile' Gestures," *People's Weekly World*, 24 June 2000, 13.

Benjamin, Phil. "Crisis Reveals Bias in Health Care Access," *Political Affairs* 11–46 (2002): 21–22.

Bertrand, Marsha. "The Cheapest Funds and the Best Funds," *Physician's Management* March (1999):18–ff.

"Dem Pol Rips Hike in Vet Health Costs," *New York Daily News*, 12 April 2005, 18.

Epstein, Deborah. "Here's Yet Another Way to Get Sued," *Medical Economics* August (2000): 35–36.

Finkelstein, Joel. "UnInsured a Problem Hard to Grasp, Solved," *AM News (NYC) Staff*, 25 April 2005.

Freking, Kevin. "Electronic Record Costs May Soar," Associated Press, 1 August 2005.

Girion, Lisa. "Don't Blame the Jury Payouts," *Los Angeles Times*, 2 June 2005.

Girion, Lisa. "Prices Accessed in Health Cost Gap," *Los Angeles Times*, 12 July 2005. www.latimes.com.

"Health Lobbyists Have Tough Sell," 29 March 2005. www.cnn.com.

Hippocrates, *The Oath*, 400 BC. Translation by Francis Adams. www.cmdik.pan.pl/zespoly/html.

ICD-9-CM Code Data Files. *Provista*, 13 July 2005. www.medical-coding.net/data/icd9/html.

Irwin, David. "Health-Care Abusers: An Untold Story," *The Monitor*, 24 April 2005.

Krueger, Alan. "Public Health Measures Always Involve Trade-Off," *Economic Scene*, 31 March 2005, 10.

Lohr, Steve. "Bush's Next Target: Malpractice Lawyers," *New York Times*, 27 February 2005.

Layton, Mary Jo. "The Doctor Is Out. Physicians Severing Ties With Insurance Plans Go It Alone," *New Jersey Times*, 19 May 2005.

Morris, David. "Bad Medicine," 10 January 2005. www.Alternet.org/story.

Nolan, Thomas, MD. "Practice Management: A Different Approach," *Physician's Management* March (1999): 1.

Pear, Robert. "Doctors in Antitrust Fight Boycott Merck Products," *New York Times,* 23 May 2000, national edition.

Preston, Susan Harrington. "Are You Being Paid Less Than You Should?" *Medical Economics* August (2000): 27–33.

Preston, Susan Harrington. "Don't Sign A Sucker Deal. Managed Care Rip-offs" *Medical Economics* August (2000): 16–23.

Reinberg, Steven. "Cutting Drug Co-Pays Lowers Costs for Insurers," *HealthDay Reporter,* 11 January 2006.

Rice, Berkeley. "Will Your HMO Pull You Through?" *Medical Economics: OB/GYN* April (1999): 66–74.

Sauders, Anne. "House Approves Changes to Small Business Health Rules," Associated Press, 30 April 2005.

Sullivan, Kip. "Invasion of Privacy," *In These Times,* 21 August 2000, 9.

Symposium. "Impact of Managed Care on Women With Cancer," *Contemporary OB/GYN* September (1999): 23–ff.

Weinstein, Steven. "Ideas & Trends: Reality Check; Will Patients' Rights Fix The Wrongs?" *New York Times Week In Review,* 24 June 2001, 1–3.

Witt, Melani, RN. "CPT Coding: What You Need To Know," *OBG Management* December (2001): *46–52.*

Zuckerman, Diana. "Hype in Medical Reporting," *Extra!,* October 2002, 8–9.

Chapter 10

"Ability to Obtain Medical Care for the Uninsured," *JAMA Study* 280:10, September 1998. http://jama/ama-assn.org/cgi/content/abstract/280/10/921.

Ackerman, Seth. "U.S. Media Favor Radical Health Reform-For Canada," *Extra!* May 2000, 7.

AFL-CIO Council Bulletin. *Vive La France. Lessons from the French Health Care System.* New Labor Forum, Summer 2003: 104–113.

Alfred, Norman, and Feldman, James. "Medical Decentralization," www.eco.utexas.edu.

Altman, Lawrence K. "Disparity in U.S. Cancer Care," *New York Times,* 16 May 2005.

"The American Health Care System Revisited," *New England Journal of Medicine,* January (1999).

American Public Health Association Bulletin. *Reforms Urged.* 30 August 2005.

Anderson, Gerard and Hussey PhD, Peter. "Health Spending in the United States and the Rest of the Industrialized World," *The Commonwealth Fund,* 2005.

Appleby, Julie. "Bush and HAS," *USA Today,* 30 January 2006. www.usatoday.com.

Barbaro, Michael. "Maryland Sets a Health Cost for Wal-Mart," *New York Times,* 13 January 2006, national edition.

"Being Uninsured: A Crisis of Income," *U.S. Newswire,* 29 August 2005.

Birdsong, Annie. "Ralph Nader and Health Care," 11 October 2000. www.wam.umd.edu.

Center for Economic and Social Rights, "Health Care as a Right," 13 November 2004, 44. www.cesr.org.

Clinton, Hillary Rodham. "Now Can We Talk About Health Care?" *New York Times Magazine,* 18 April 2004, 26-30.

Clift, Eleanor. "It's Big-Issue Time," *MSNBC* (web exclusive commentary), 16 December 2005. www.msnbc.com.

Connolly, Ceci. "Religion-Linked Hospitals Accused of Price-Gouging Uninsured," *Washington Post,* 28 August 2005.

Conyers, John. HR 676, *The Congressional Record* (11 February 2003).

Costello, Daniel. "Ethical Hang-ups Over Dial-A-Doc," *Health Today am New York,* 21 November 2005, 24.

Cusac, Anne-Marie. "Cut Loose. Companies Trick Retirees Out of Health Benefits," *The Progressive,* April (2001), 21–22.

Dalrymple, Mary. "House, Senate Republicans Work on the Budget," The Associated Press, 26 April 2005.

Dellums, Ronald. "HR 1374, A Bill," 17 April 1997.

Department of Health. Press Notice. 30 September 2002. 2220/0241.

Dohenny, Kathleen. "Access to Mammography On the Decline," *Health Day,* 28 April 2005. www.healthdaynews.com.

Drummond, Hugh, MD. "Take Two Echocardiograms and Call Me In the Morning," *Mother Jones,* November 1986, 17–20.

Espo, David. "House Deems Proposing Health Care Agenda," The Associated Press, 3 May 2005.

Farrell, Chris. "It's Time to Cure Health Care," *SoundMoney, Businessweek,* 23 January 2006.

Finkelstein, Katherina. "Rebels in White Coats" *Utne Reader,* from The Nation, May/June 2000.

"Fix the Prescriptions," *The Progressive,* 8 August 2004. www.progressive.org.

Fox, Maggie. "Study of Racism in U.S. Health Care System," Reuters, 19 July 2005.

Frosch, Dan. "Your Money or Your Life," *Nation,* 21 February 2005, 11–12.

Green, Jennie. "What's Health Care, Mom?" 12 November 2003. http://www.alternet.com.

"The Health and Productivity Cost of the Top Ten Physical and Mental Health Conditions," *Journal of Occupational and Environmental Medicine* (2006). www.joem.org/pt/re/joem/abstract.00043764-200301000-00007.htm.

Himmelstein MD, Davi and Woolhandler MD, Stephanie. "The Corporate Compromise and Marxist View of Health Maintenance Organizations," *Annals of Internal Medicine, American College of Physicians* September (1988): 494–501.

Himmelstein MD, David, and Woolhandler MD, Stephanie. "Cure a Sick Healthcare System," *In These Times,* 6 August 2004, 32–ff.

Himmelstein MD, David, and Woolhandler MD, Stephanie. "U.S. Health Reform: Unkindest Cuts," *The Nation,* 22 January 1996, 16–20.

HR 676, 108th Congress. *Congressional Record 11* (February 2003).

Jackson, Derrick. "As Goes General Motors," Globe Newspaper Company, 19 October 2005.

Kaczocha, Paul. "HR 676. Everybody In, Nobody Out," *PWW,* 2 February 2004, 14.

Kass, Leon. "Lingering Longer: Who Would Care?" *American Enterprise Institute Bulletin,* 29 September 2005.

Kling, Arnold. "Health Insurance and Bankruptcy," *Bookmark,* 2 February 2005.

Kling, Arnold. "The Myth of Massive Health Care Waste," *TCS Tech Central Station,* 21 March 2005.

Krugman, Paul. "Ailing Health Care," OpEd, *New York Times,* 1 April 2005, national edition.

Krugman, Paul. "Pride, Prejudice, Insurance," OpEd, *New York Times,* 7 November 2005, national edition.

LeBow MD, Robert. "Health Care Meltdown," *Alan C Hood Co.*, 2004.

Levy, Marc. "Blacks Less Likely to Have Health Insurance," Associated Press, 10 May 2005.

Lovett, Kenneth. "HMO Premiums Soaring," *New York Post*, 7 September 2005.

Lueck, Sarah and John McKinnon. "Bush Focus on Health Care," *Wall Street Journal*, 12 January 2006.

Lutton, Linda. "A Healthy Choice. Health Care as a Basic Right. The Bernardin Agreement," *In These Times*, 2 May 1999, 9.

Medical Data International. HMO Penetration by State. 2005. www.medicaldata.com.

Moffit PhD, Robert, and Christina Sochhacki. "The Promise of Personalized Health Care" *WebMemo #801*, 20 July 2005.

Moy, Chelsi. "Health Insurance Pool OK'd," *Helena, Montana Gazette State Bureau*, 16 April 2005.

National Economic and Social Rights Initiative. (NESRI). *Human Right to Health*. Info Sheet HI.

Nelson, Joyce. "NAFTA's Bitter Pill," *Z Magazine*, May 1995, 18.

Olson, Karen. "The Greening of Health Care," *Utne*, November 2002, 85. www.utne.com.

Parenti, Christian. "U.S. Healthcare, The Free Choice to Suck," 27 June 2003. www.altertnet.org.

"Patient-Physician Racial Concordance and the Perceived Quality and Use of Healthcare," *JAMA Study*, 159:9 (May 1999). http://archinte.ama-assn.org/cgi/content/abstract/159/9/997.

Pear, Robert. "U.S. Gives Florida a Sweeping Right to Curb Medicaid," *New York Times*, 30 October 2005, national edition.

Rauber, Chris. "Medicare Madness," *San Francisco Business Times*, 23 October 2005. www.medicaremadness_sanfransisco_msnbc.com.

Schneider, Mary Ellen. "Poor Health of Uninsured Carries High Price Tag," *ObGyn News*, August (2003): 25–26.

Shalala, Donna. "Needed: Fast Federal Action," *The Washington Post*, 26 September 2005.

Sullivan, Kip. "Rationing Health Care Is Not Necessary. It Is Unethical and Wrong," *Z Magazine*, May 2001, 41-44.

Terry, Ken. "What's In the Box? Is United Healthcare Delivering On Its Promises," *Medical Economics* October 2000: 120–ff.

Top 10 Issues for the HealthCare Industry in 2006, PriceWaterhouseCoopers (PRWEB), 10 January 2006. www.pwc.com.

U.S. Department of Labor Subtopics. *Employee Retirement Income Security.* Act-ERISA. 9 May 2005.

Vardi, Nathan. "Moore's Law," *Forbes,* 28 November 2005, 116-120.

Von Zielbauer, Paul. "As Health Care in Jails Goes Private, 10 Days Can Be a Death Sentence," *New York Times,* 27 February 2005, national edition.

Warren, Elizabeth. et al, "A Double Whammy for Americans' Health," *The Baltimore Sun,* 12 May 2005.

"Wrong Fix for Health Care; Local Laws Won't Solve National Problem," *Newsday,* 3 Oct 2005.

Zuger, Abigail. "Lavish Care by "Boutique Doctors," *New York Times,* 30 October 2005, national edition.

INDEX

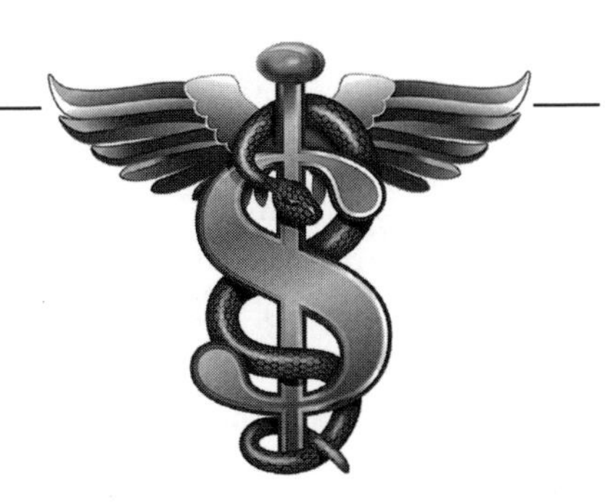

Other Titles from Caveat Press

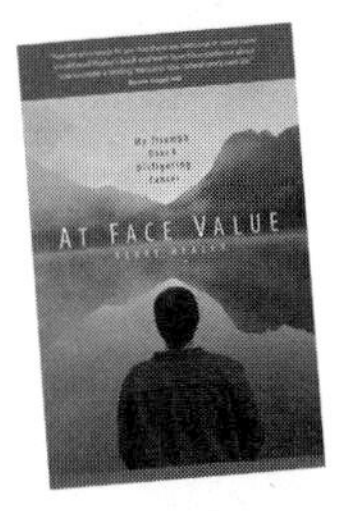

At Face Value: My Triumph Over A Disfiguring Cancer
by Terry Healey
ISBN: 1-883991-98-6 / Paperback: $16.95

The Death of Mammography: How Our Best Defense Against Breast Cancer Is Being Driven to Extinction
by René Jackson, RN, BSN, MS and Alberto Righi, MD
ISBN: 0-9745245-3-0 / Paperback: $19.95

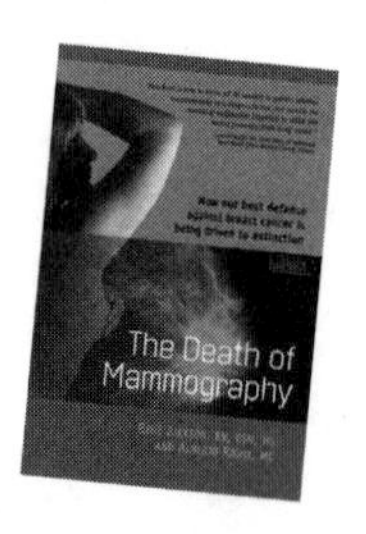

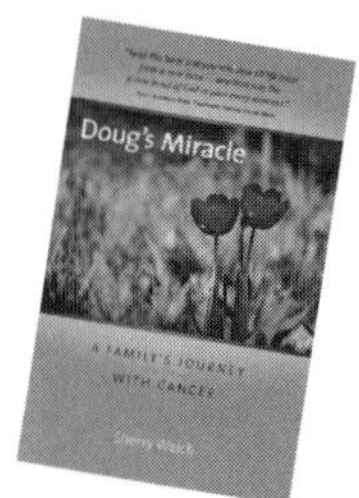

Doug's Miracle: A Family's Journey with Cancer
by Sherry Welch
ISBN: 0-9745245-1-4 / Paperback: $14.95

Maximum Fitness Minimum Risk: The Wellness Exercise Program for Cardiac, Diabetes, and Pulmonary Patients
by Carole Marshall
ISBN: 0-9745245-0-6 / Paperback: $16.9

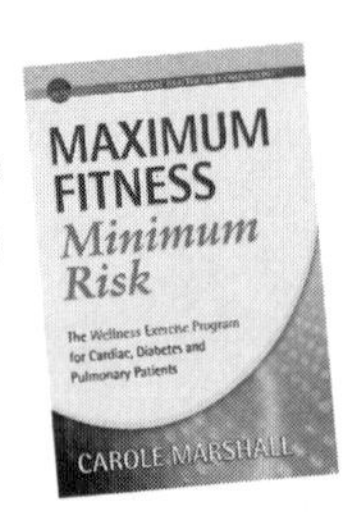

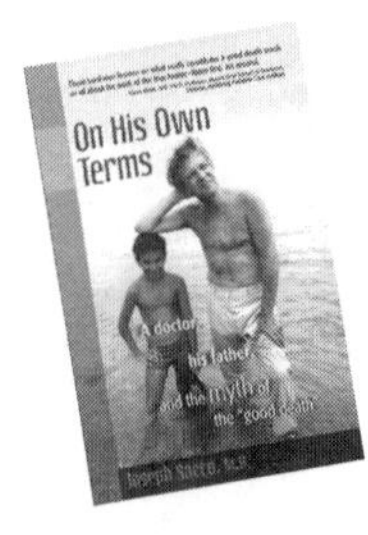

On His Own Terms: A Doctor, His Father, and the Myth of the "Good Death"
by Joseph Sacco, MD
ISBN: 0-9745245-2-2 / Paperback: $14.95

One Trip Around the Sun: A Guide to Using Diet, Herbs, Exercise, and Meditation to Harmonize with the Seasons
by Rory Lipsky, LAc
ISBN: 1-883991-85-4 / Paperback: $19.95

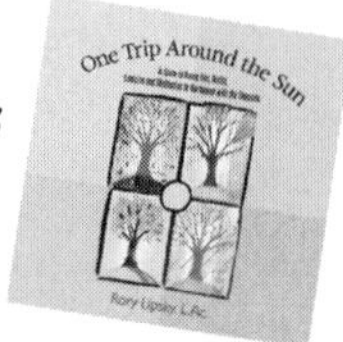